My Marathon:
Winning the race against an eating disorder

Jesse Harmon

Thanks for the support!

II Cor. 5:17

Contents

Pre-race

2:58

That was it. I did it. All the hard work I had put in finally came to fruition. I met my goal and ran a marathon under three hours. Now it was done. I crossed the finish line with arms held high, received my medal, and told my family, "We're going to Disney World!"

It was the Jacksonville Bank marathon in December 2012. I trained for an entire year to run my three-hour goal, and I had done it. In my book, I had won.

But it didn't come easy. Goals are met through hard work, dedicated time and effort, and lots of patience from others, especially my family. I decided in December of 2011 that I wanted to set the goal: to run a marathon under three hours. I started training in January, gradually building my speed and endurance for the race. If there's one thing I've learned about running is that speed *and* endurance don't come easy. Sure running itself is hard, but what's harder is the patience it requires. Big results take continuous work, and continuous work takes patience--and a lot of it!

2012 was full of small goals. I trained throughout the year, running shorter races to try and gauge where I was physically by the numbers. In running, the numbers don't lie. The lower the number, the better you are. The shorter your time, the better your fitness. That's the way most runners live. And it soon became the way I lived too. No matter how good I felt during a run, the numbers told the "truth." And if the numbers showed me I was slower than the day before, that meant the run was bad--no matter how I felt. The numbers determined everything.

I ran well all year. I ran faster than I had ever run before. However, I began to enjoy the training less as I focused on the numbers more. At times, running felt like an obligation-- something I had to do. I would catch myself thinking that if I skipped a run, my fitness level would go down, I would gain weight, and then lose everything I had worked so hard to obtain. Looking back, I now know none of that was true. What my body was telling me was that it needed and wanted rest, nourishment, and time to recharge. But at the time, I kept my foot on the gas pedal and continued training.

During training I had everything I needed. I had a Garmin watch that would update me on all my split times and a scale to monitor my weight so I knew I was keeping myself in the best fitness of my life (at least that's what I thought).

I evaluated my running by the numbers. But without even realizing it, I slowly began to evaluate other areas of my life by the numbers.

Weight is a topic of concentration for distance runners. Runners talk about reaching their "race weight," that ideal weight that will help them perform their best on race day. The theory behind it is this: the lighter you are, the faster you can be. The goal is to find the "perfect" weight for you to perform at your best. Not a bad idea in theory, but it can be dangerous when put into practice without proper nutrition guidance. Lighter is not always better. Lighter does not always mean faster. We are all created different; no one person is alike. There is no cookie cutter mold for a fast runner. Each person is given a different body to operate.

My struggle came when my mind slowly began to convince me that I needed to be lighter to be faster. Lighter *can* mean faster, but only when it isn't sacrificing muscle mass and overall health. Muscle is what propels us forward. If we begin to lose weight because of muscle loss then we become a slower, more unhealthy person.

For me, the goal was to get lower--not healthier. My focus became cloudy and the priority of a lower weight became paramount. The lower my weight, the faster my runs. And the faster my runs, the lower my times. Numbers. I stopped focusing on the things I knew to be true of health and fitness and started to focus only on the number on my scale.

And soon the numbers really did rule everything. 2012 was a great year according to the numbers, but it was a slow fade into an addiction and disease that would come close to taking my life.

The account in this book is not to offer advice for someone dealing with addictions, eating disorders or any other obsessive behaviors. It's simply to give an inside look into my life and how anorexia affected me and the people around me. My hope is to let those battling with eating disorders and addictions know that you are not alone and recovery *is* possible.

MILE

I

How the race began

Goals are good. I worked for an entire year for this event: the 2012 Jacksonville Bank Marathon. Marathons can be very intimidating mentally. You train for a long time for one day, one race. Everything is put under a microscope. During a marathon, when the smallest thing goes wrong it could derail your race day goals and nullify all your hard work. All scenarios are playing in your head as you prep for race day. The nervousness is part of the fun. It's part of the sport. You know you've trained and worked hard to get to the start line but you don't know how the race will go.

I didn't start entering running events until I was 24. I was a recreational runner up until that point. I would run a 2-3 mile loop around my house or campus, but never took anything seriously. I never had any organized running plans, workouts, or goals. It wasn't until the local gym hosted a 5k that I got the bug for running.

At 24 years old I ran a 5k as a newly married, weightlifting, 185-pound guy. My wife ran cross-country in high school and a little in college, and when we first met we would go on summer runs together. I remember how nervous I was the first time we ran together. I knew I had to be on my A game because I was running with a college athlete. On our first run, my goal was to keep up with her. I had to maintain her pace; I couldn't let her outrun me. I just knew if she would outrun me then she would just keep running until she found another guy. I gave it all I had to keep up, and luckily that first run I was able to hold my own long enough to get her to stick around. Praise God!

Running my first 5k was an incredible experience. I had set a goal of running seven minutes per mile. I wanted to see if I could reach my goal so I worked hard towards that time. I had no clue how to prepare for a 5k. I figured I would first have to get use to running three miles without stopping, and so I tried everything to do just that. I went to the local track and wore weight vests, ankle weights, and anything else I could find. I figured if I could run with 15 pound weights on me then running without them would be easier, right? Well, that's true but running on a track with a weight vest isn't pleasant. I blistered my back and stomach from the friction of the vest rubbing against me. I can only imagine the spectacle I gave other people who were also on the track. I did notice that more and more people would seem to show up around the track each time I did a workout. Looking back I wonder if my getup had anything to do with the growth in attendance?

I wasn't sure what was going to happen when it actually came time to run that first race. I remember the anxiety about what to wear, how early I should arrive, and how much and what I should eat. All legitimate concerns, right? The day came and went without incident. I ran the race, met my goal, and enjoyed the entire experience. Well, I say the entire experience. As runners entered the parking lot to finish the race, there was an ambulance parked at the exit. I remember passing by and feeling like I should just collapse and let them handle it from there. It was all extremely painful yet rewarding at the same time.

As soon as I got back home I wanted to find another one and race again, but what came next? I had no idea where to look for additional races or what other distances were offered. Looking through many websites I found a 10k (6.2 miles) through a web search that was about a month away. I had no idea where to set my goal. I didn't know how to train for a 10k. What was I supposed to do to run 6.2 miles? I decided to just set a goal to try and run a 10k at the same pace I just ran a 5k.

Well, that 10k did not go as planned. It was one of the most painful experiences to date in my life. Apparently, this race found every mountain (very small hill that felt like a mountain) in the Lexington and West Columbia area. I found out later that the local kids call one of the hills "thrill hill" because of how steep the decline is. Just my luck! However, no matter how painful the experience, I loved every step. It was official; I was hooked!

Soon after I set the big goal: I wanted to run a marathon. Sometimes people confuse the meaning of the word marathon. Just to be clear, a marathon is a race distance that equals 26.2 miles. I'm a big picture kind of guy. I want to know the highest peak, the toughest challenge. I wanted to set an achievable goal and pursue it. I had been running only a few months. While I didn't know much about the sport, I knew that I loved how it made me feel. So I registered for my first marathon in March of 2007!

My wife is the levelheaded one in our family. She cautioned me about doing a marathon before running a half marathon. She really didn't understand this newfound love of running in me, but she did understand me. She knew that when I become focused on something, I was bound and determined to complete it. I was always going to give it my best. So in this case, she knew that the best thing to do was just sit back, watch (maybe laugh), and cheer me on!

So I became focused on the marathon. I began to love running. I would research how to get faster, what to eat, how to hydrate, what types of shoes to buy, and so much more. I wasn't educated on the sport but wanted to learn as much as I could. My initial marathon training consisted of long runs, usually anything more than 12 miles for me. Now 12 miles is nothing to laugh at when less than a year ago I wasn't even running half that distance in one run.

In other words, I needed a plan. I researched the internet and found one that would help me gain the needed fitness and leg strength to finish a 26.2-mile race. I followed the plan as closely as I could. I wanted to be prepared as possible. However, the more I trained, the less I could fathom actually running 26.2 miles! Still, I pressed on.

Throughout my training there were a variety of runs. Sometimes I would do a faster five-mile run, and sometimes I did speedwork around a track. The speedwork sessions were very painful. Consisting of shorter intervals around a track, speedwork sessions had me doing at least one or two laps at an incredibly fast pace. There were times when I couldn't feel my arms, felt like I was going to throw up, and found myself faced with the infamous side stitch! However, there was a sense of satisfaction after I realized I wasn't going to die. I was getting better... slowly but surely.

A must for marathon training, I scheduled long runs every other Saturday. Gradually, my long runs lengthened to 20 miles. I remember the first time I ran 20 miles. I mapped my route to finish at the church where I worked because I thought if I was going to die, it might as well be on the church grounds! After finishing my first 20-mile run, I knew there would be no chance of walking the next day. I was sore and kept getting worse by the minute. Lying in bed that night, I remember thinking that I might not wake up in the morning. That's how bad it hurt. I didn't see how my body could handle so much pain. Thankfully, it did! Even though I was suffering, there was a sense of accomplishment with each mile completed. I gained confidence in my ability to accomplish goals when I worked hard.

I slowly progressed toward marathon day, and then suddenly, that day arrived. I finally made it, and I had no clue what to feel. I was nervous, scared, excited... just about every emotion you could imagine. I had worked hard to get here and was ready for that hard work to pay off. The only problem? It was freezing on race morning. I grew up in South Carolina for a reason; it's cold for about three weeks during winter, and that was it. Because of that, most of race morning consisted of me trying to figure out how to stay warm. Forget all the stretching, and warm ups; I wanted hot chocolate! My body temperature slowly rose during the race only after running with my hands in my pants for the first three miles to keep them from falling off.

I ran and enjoyed every second. A key thing I learned in running that race is that there is nothing longer on earth than the last 6.2 miles of a marathon. The distance may only display as 6.2 miles but the feeling your body goes through makes it seem more like 600.2! I gutted my way through my first marathon and crossed the finish line proud as can be. I've always made fun of people who sprint through the finish chute as if they want others to believe that they somehow ran that fast during the entire race. However, in this race, I was that guy. My wife filmed me as I ran the final portion of the race, and I was running as fast as I could. I wanted to impress those watching. In my mind I knew I was at least running a sub six-minute mile, but my form had to look like that of an experienced Kenyan runner. However, when I watched the video my wife took of me running over the finish line I remember thinking, "I'm barely moving!"

I finished second in my age group in my first marathon. As I crossed the finish line, the flood of memories and emotions of middle school returned. The times where I felt a need to fit in, a desire to be skinny, and was made fun of for being overweight. None of it mattered. Everyone that made a point to comment on my weight and the feelings of seclusion I felt were tossed out the window. I'll talk more about my early life experiences later in the book. I was able to rise above all of those negative thoughts and sayings because now, I was a marathon finisher.

The exhilaration of completing a marathon is huge but adding finishing so well for your age only intensified the excitement. To hold the marathon medal in my hand and relive all the long runs, hard work, and dedication I put into training gave me a sense of accomplish. It was like a new identity, and it felt good. It's a feeling I wish for everyone.

My first marathon I finished in 3:31:48--just a few seconds per mile off my goal pace. It didn't matter though because I had a blast. And I wanted to run more. I went back home and looked for upcoming marathons. What could be next? When could I run again?

My goals have always progressed. After that first race, each marathon became a little faster for me. My second marathon was in Charlotte in 2007. That one was painful. I finished faster but barely, clocking in at 3:26. Then I knew I wanted to try to qualify for Boston. The Boston Marathon is *the* event for us casual runners. It's like our Olympics. It's a race that you have to qualify for prior to the run. That's not an easy task, but I wanted to try. I thought if I could qualify, it would solidify me as a real runner. My qualifying time was 3:10, meaning I now had to complete a marathon in less than 3 hours 10 minutes to be accepted into the Boston race. Well, third time's the charm for me: 3:08:19. I qualified for Boston at the Kiawah Island Marathon in 2009, just about three years after I started running.

I ran the Boston Marathon in April of 2011. Looking back I wish I had enjoyed it more. I had put a little time into training but hadn't been as hyper focused as I had for prior races. I wanted this race to be more of a fun marathon. Plus, Sarah and I had our first child in January of that year so my training schedule was a little off to say the least.

After Boston I took a little time off and tried to figure out what my next goal would be. I ran a few races in the fall and then decided that I wanted to try to break three hours in a marathon the following year. This new goal brought a rekindled passion to train and focus on running. Without a race or goal in mind, running can be painful and boring. I've found I need a goal to keep me going and motivated.

So I made a one-year plan. I had goals that I tried to meet throughout the year to help me build my fitness level along the way. My first goal was to run a personal best in a 5k race in May. My 5k times are very pedestrian for the semi-serious runners; I just wasn't made to be a 5k guy! My legs don't turnover that fast. However, I was able to muster the mojo on that day and run a new PR, besting my goal time. I was both happy and relieved!

Slowly, everything started to focus around my performance, and that isn't necessarily a bad thing. Performance focus helped me eat healthier, sleep better, and be overall a healthier person. But along the way, I started noticing how much easier running was when I was lighter. As my weight decreased, I associated my faster running times with this new, lighter me. Weight gain slowly began to consume my mind. I started to weigh in multiple times a day. Eating began to bring a new fear--a fear that I didn't understand but remembered from my childhood. It was a fear of gaining weight. If I gained the weight, I couldn't run as fast. If I couldn't run as fast, I would lose my identity. Everything I had worked so hard for would be gone.

By September of 2012 my weight was down to approx. 135 pounds. I was still consuming about 2000 calories a day, but most of my calories came in just breakfast and dinner. I didn't like to eat lunch because it was just me. Sarah worked as a teacher during the day, and I worked from home at the time. I wanted to share meals with my wife so I typically skipped lunch. And besides, I didn't understand how I could eat three meals a day and feel great. My thoughts had shifted to only eating two meals a day. If I did eat three meals then I had to run twice.

Thus began a season of disordered eating in my life. Disordered eating is different than an eating disorder in that disordered eating is more about developing abnormal eating behaviors. The main difference between the two is the level of severity and the frequency of the eating habits. Along with this, I did constant mental calculations of calories throughout the day. But I was still training hard and performing very well. Even though my eating habits had changed, they hadn't begun to take an effect on my performance. Looking back, I think that's because of the years of quality nutrition and muscle mass I had developed.

By December, I was 128 pounds. From August on, I dropped seven pounds. That amount of weight factors to be a little more than a pound a month which isn't that drastic, but the food choices I was making were horrible. I started to look at carbs as bad, only eating them prior to a run. Grilled chicken salad was the staple of my diet. At this point I was pretty familiar with what I needed to eat and drink to lose weight. I reached 128 pounds approximately three weeks before the marathon and had run well so I thought that would be the best weight for me. As race day drew near I went into full preparation mode. Two days before the event I consumed only 800 calories a day. There wasn't really a rhyme or reason to it. It's what I did during training that resulted in good runs at the time so I thought it would now as well. Plus, if I didn't run as much, I couldn't eat as much.

My family and I were both excited and relieved that marathon day had arrived. I ran the race of my life. I had put in hours of preparation getting ready for the event, and my intentions were always good. There's nothing wrong with the aspiration of running a fast marathon. There's nothing wrong with setting goals as a runner to perform better, run faster, and train harder. But the methods I was using to do so were detrimental and dangerous. I just didn't know it yet.

2:58:42. I was able to run that fast for a marathon because I was the lightest I had ever been. That's what I believed. There may be a very small percentage of truth in that, but the larger percentage of truth is this: I was unhealthy. I was not a strong runner. That day happened because of years of strength training, good nutrition, and hard work. It wasn't because I was skinny.

128 pounds.

Six years earlier I married a beautiful woman, and I was 185 pounds. I dropped close to 60 pounds in six years. That averages close to a pound per month since my marriage. Please understand that is in no way a reflection of my wife's cooking. She is a great cook! That low weight came from nutrition decisions that seemed innocent at the time. But soon, they took control of my life.

Post Race

Sometimes it's hard to explain how I feel after a great race. This was the case for me the day of the Jacksonville Bank Marathon. I'd had so much fun. I'd put in so much work. And it had all paid off. The feelings were so satisfying. While I was glad it was over, I was left wondering: now what?

I had trained for an entire year for just one race. I knew it was time to rest, to enjoy the extra time with family, and take it easy for a while. But some things are easier said than done.

As a runner, I was so focused on my race goal. And I loved it! The challenged inspired me. And the thought of suddenly having no race on the calendar to work towards-- no challenge to rise and meet--was not easy to face.

As the news spread that day to friends and family that I had completed my race, the congratulations came pouring in. And along with them, this instruction: "Great! Now go eat a cheeseburger!"

This half-hearted comment had become a common phrase during my journey. Throughout my training, my weight had dropped to an all-time low. It wasn't because I didn't eat. In fact, it was just the opposite. I was eating all the time, but only more of the lower calorie foods. I stayed well aware of the nutrition facts of every food I ate. I would research calorie amounts. Caloric restriction paired with running all the time caused a steady weight loss. Most of my days beginning in August of 2012 consisted of two runs a day. I would do a morning run and evening run, totaling 12 to 15 miles per day.

As we went back to our hotel after the Jacksonville race, thoughts of life post-race came into my mind. I knew logically that I needed to take a few days off from running, but I honestly didn't want to, In my mind, a few days off from running meant a few days behind on my fitness. But it also meant I couldn't eat.

On days that I didn't run I would restrict my diet to around 1,000 calories. Somehow I was convinced that's what I needed to do not to gain weight. I hated rest days. Eating and food were things I looked forward to, and on non-run days, I could do neither. I knew if I didn't run I would lose my fitness. I know that might sound silly, but I had worked so hard. I didn't want to lose it all! I also knew that I would have to go home and weigh. I knew the scale was waiting on me, and I didn't want to see the number. Everything I ate--every time I swallowed--I could hear the voice saying, "Don't eat that; you are going to gain weight!"

That's how it started. It was a small thought really, but I realize now how big the repercussions would be. If I couldn't eat normal, I couldn't run. Normal meant three meals a day with adequate caloric intake, and I couldn't do that unless I was running. If I did, I would gain weight, and I thought I would be miserable. Where I found my identity was starting to change. How I enjoyed life was beginning to change.

My life soon became consumed by the scale, food, and running. If I'm not running, I need to eat less, I thought.

To me, it seemed logical. I wanted to maintain my level of fitness and weight over the next few days without running. In order to do this I would have to restrict what I was eating.

In my recovery I learned where this fear of losing fitness and gaining weight came from. It was really a fear of losing control over an area of my life. Running allowed me to eat guilt free, and that was something I didn't experience a child. Back then, eating was filled with a temporary satisfaction followed by a tremendous amount of guilt. I would overeat, and the guilt, even though temporary, was very painful and loud. So it was during my times of rest from running that this fear started to creep back in and tried to take over my life.

The night of the Jacksonville race we went to one of our favorite restaurants to kick off the post-race celebration: Cheesecake Factory. There, I ordered my regular order: a salad and dessert. Salad may seem like a diet food to some, but I eat salad based on taste. I order a salad with all the goods on it. I want the cheese, the bacon, as much meat as they will give me, and all the sauces to go along with it! I don't want any sort of low calorie dressing. I want it all!

That meal was all a mental game. All I could think about while I was eating was that I wouldn't run for three days so I shouldn't be eating this food. You would think I would be able to eat anything I wanted because I just ran a marathon, but that was not the case.

It was a struggle to eat any of the dessert. Each bite brought feelings of guilt, my thoughts screaming, "Don't do it! You're not running tomorrow!" This was supposed to be a celebration. I had just accomplished a goal I never thought possible, but I was frustrated with feelings over my weight.

The few days after the marathon, the family and I headed to Disney World to celebrate. The idea of eating that elusive cheeseburger was hovering in the back of my mind. But along with it, a new thought: I don't have another run planned so I shouldn't eat it. I couldn't eat. Every time I thought about eating, I instantly was hit with the thought of having to weigh in when I got home. What would the scale say after that cheeseburger?

It wasn't that I was concerned with gaining the weight back--at least that's what I kept telling myself. But the thought of gaining weight consumed me. My obsessive tendencies now were completely fixated on my weight. I'd worked so hard to get to this point as a runner that I didn't want to ruin my progress by gaining weight. I had created a new identity, one that was engulfed in running and performance. I couldn't lose it now. I couldn't gain weight. That's how I associated losing progress: gaining weight.

The idea of maintaining fitness in and of itself isn't bad but the measures I took to maintain weight or to lose weight were damaging to my body and overall health. Without even realizing it, I had begun to associate maintaining my level of fitness with avoiding weight gain at all costs. If you are eating healthy, consuming the right amount of calories, and properly maintaining hydration then maintaining your weight is a very healthy way to live. My weight maintenance was not healthy and didn't focus on feeding my body the proper foods. The only way I knew to avoid sabotaging my hard work was to start carefully limiting what I ate and drank in order to know how many calories I consumed every meal.

I needed a plan.

But more than that, I needed to run.

I didn't change my diet to reflect extreme changes right away. At first, they were simply good decisions to improve my overall health. For example, I tried to reduce or avoid fried foods. Eating deep fried food isn't good for the overall cholesterol anyway. But slowly, over the course of years I would continue to take specific foods out of my diet in hopes that it would help improve my running economy. Please understand, none of my diet changes were monitored or suggested by a certified nutritionist. The changes were only based on what I thought would improve my running. I had very limited knowledge of health and nutrition at the time.

Mile

2

Eddie

As I continued losing weight and becoming a faster runner memories of my childhood would rear their ugly head and come back to haunt me. This is where the disease started to get an unbelievable grip on me. Soon, I met Eddie. Eddie controlled my life. He had me always focused on the numbers. The watch, the scale, everything that had a number--Eddie had me monitoring it like a hawk. I was obsessed with the number on the scale. I had everything calculated that I did during my day. I knew everything that would lower the number on the scale or get me back to the number I thought I needed to be. There was no way I could have run that fast without being 128 pounds. There was no way I could come close to breaking three hours without being at or close to that weight.

At least that's what Eddie would tell me. Those were his lies.

Who in the world is Eddie? Another child? Parent? Friend?

No, Eddie is an acronym for eating disorder. During counseling I was advised to give my disorder a name. After all, he is real; in actuality, he influenced my decisions, thought processes, and direction. So I named him Eddie (born from the acronym for eating disorder). Clever, I know.

Eddie is not an audible voice that I hear speaking to me. He's more of the subtle feeling, a whisper. It's frustrating because even though he's not a tangible person, he's very believable. He has convinced me of things that I knew were not true about my health and food. Coupled with my weight obsession, Eddie had very destructive consequences on my life.

Eddie is that voice I heard in middle school that convinced me that I was the fattest person in the class. The voice that I listened to that said I wasn't as athletic as the other guys because I wasn't skinny. Eddie also convinced me I couldn't fit in or do what I wanted in life because of my weight. Eddie would tell me that other people's perception of me was that I was lazy, unable to be good at anything because I was bigger.

Well, I set out to prove Eddie wrong. I wanted to be fit and in shape. I wanted to show Eddie that I wasn't always going to be fat. I could be skinny and make something of myself. I had something to prove.

Little did I know I would keep hearing from Eddie for a long time in my life. He was always there, ready to remind me of my lack of self-confidence. He would say, "Remember, you're only happy because you're in shape." He would use positive reinforcement as a way to let me know he was still there, whispering things like, "See, I told you. You are skinnier now and having fun. You have a girlfriend all because you are skinny. If you want it to last, you have to stay skinny." All of those things are lies; I see that now. But I believed them for a long time.

Eddie has been laying the foundation for an obsessive focus on my body for as long as I can remember. He was there in seventh grade when a girl sitting behind me in class made sure I know that I was, in her opinion, the fattest kid in class. I'd been one of the bigger kids since elementary school, but I'd never heard anyone say it aloud. Eddie continued to compound my sense of largeness in seventh grade through a humiliating experience running the mile. I'd experienced this same humiliation in elementary school (which I'll share more on as the story unfolds), but the embarrassment continued into middle school. It wasn't until I had a breakthrough during my freshmen year of high school running the mile that Eddie convinced me running could be my ticket to freedom.

Mile

3

Life as a roadrunner

Running wasn't always a passion of mine. In fact, it actually started out as more of a fear.

Growing up in rural Lexington, South Carolina, there weren't many places to stay active outside of joining local community sports leagues. I mean there were tons of open fields and places to play, but nothing really organized. There weren't streetlights to let kids stay out after dark and play. When the sun went down, we went inside. That was that.

My family lived in Lexington all of my life. My mom owned her own business while my dad worked for a distribution metal company. I attended Red Bank Elementary until sixth grade (how ironic that our school mascot was a roadrunner, Go Roadrunners!). Life was simple, and I liked it that way.

Throughout most of my childhood, I was noticeably identified as the "big kid" because I was on the heavier side. Fortunately for me, I was also one of the tallest. Being both helped cover the fact that I was essentially overweight. It made it easier to find ways to hide it. I didn't like tight clothes. If clothes were loose then it would cover up any of the fat I had. And I didn't want people to ever fully know I was overweight.

It was frustrating to be the "big kid." Of course it came with stereotypes, the most frustrating of which being that because I was overweight, I couldn't be athletic. I loved sports. I have always been an avid South Carolina fan and loved playing basketball with the neighbors. But it seemed like I was always picked last for kickball games, the last name to be called to join a group in PE, and just generally avoided when it came to anything athletic. And each time, I was more and more frustrated. I remember thinking, "You're wrong! I am athletic! Pick me and I'll prove it!" I had the motivation to work hard and prove myself; I just needed the opportunity to do it.

And that's where Eddie would come in, saying things like, "Man, it's because you are overweight. If only you were skinny, then you'd get picked. Those other kids out there are skinnier and faster than you. That's why they were picked before you." The truth is, whenever there's a group of kids and everyone is picked one by one, someone is going to get picked last. But Eddie was giving me a reason why I was picked last. And even though it sounds silly, I believed it. Of course I didn't realize at the time that what I was feeling then would lead to an eating disorder, but looking back, I can see Eddie's impact on my self-perception and confidence started even then.

Anyone who struggled with weight in their youth can understand the feelings of seclusion, separation, and frustration that come with being labeled the "big kid." It's almost as if you can feel the looks and comments that other people are making. I always thought it was ironic because people would say them to me as if being bigger was something I liked--something that couldn't possibly bother me. Of course it bothered me! I tried to cover it up by joking around, figuring that if I could somehow show others it didn't bother me, then they would actually think I was fine with it. Not even close.

I remember lying in bed at night just wishing that I could be a skinny kid. Skinny kids just seemed to fit in; they never got noticed for the negative things about them. To me, they were normal, and I didn't think I could ever be seen as normal if I was already being seen as the "big kid." I couldn't define myself because my weight already defined me.

These feelings of isolation in my childhood laid the foundation for the fear that crept in later in my life. I didn't want to go back to being the "big kid." And Eddie used that fear to remind me never to gain weight. "Do whatever you have to do not to gain weight," he would say. I was afraid that if I gained just one pound, it would be the first step towards another and another. So I couldn't gain any weight--not even one pound.

Life as the "big kid" developed in me an unspoken belief that I would never amount to much more than that. In my mind, my weight limited my potential. And because I didn't know how to be anyone other than the "big kid," I would never be anything else.

That couldn't be farther from the truth.

When someone says something about you or you have feelings of self doubt, stop and ask yourself this question: "Where's the truth in that?"

For example not being picked for a game of pickup kickball would make me think, "they don't want me on their team because I'm fat kid." Says who? How do I know that' true? Did someone tell me that? Not at all! There was no truth in the things I believed were motivating them to make their decisions. Eddie had convinced me to believe in lies.

Mile

4

The mile

It was in fifth grade that our PE teacher introduced the mile run fitness test. While some considered it a fun way to help kids evaluate their own health, as an overweight fifth grader, I considered it pure torture. My teacher should have just asked us to climb Mt. Everest because to me both seemed to take the same amount of energy. How in the world was I going to run a mile... in front of my peers?

I was completely intimidated. The most I'd run up to that point was a meek three laps around the bases during baseball practice. The thought of actually running an entire mile left me nauseated. The scary part for me was that even if some of my classmates didn't recognize that I was the fattest kid in the class then they definitely would now. I knew I was athletic. I believed I was athletic, but everyone else thought I wasn't. There was no way I would finish ahead of many of the other kids. I wasn't in good shape at all, but the mile would prove exactly what I believed all my classmates were thinking: he's fat, slow, and unathletic.

Unfortunately there was no getting out of it. That mile was for a grade, and everyone had to participate. The date was set, and there was nothing I could do but begin my mental preparation for the pain and embarrassment that was sure to come.

As I arrived to class the day of the mile run, I lingered in the back as the coach went over our instructions. Students were to pair up and take turns running the mile while a partner kept count of your laps. When the last lap was completed, the partner was to alert the PE coach who would then yell out your final time for the mile. Then she detailed the route: 13 laps around the basketball blacktop.

Thirteen laps?! She might as well have said 1,300 because in my mind there was no way I could do that many laps. I remember eyeing the blacktop, trying to compare it to my only previous running experience on the baseball diamond. At baseball practice our coach would make us run three laps around the bases, and I would always feel like I was going to throw up. Now I have to run 13? I wasn't much of a praying man then, but I sure started praying. I needed a miracle. I needed some wings or a strong tailwind-- anything that would help! From where I was standing, it definitely looked bigger than a baseball field. I was in trouble.

Time came to select our lap partner, and as usual, mine was tough to find. No one wanted to run the mile with the "big kid." You would think this would be my infamous time of popularity. Here's your chance to run with the slow guy. There's no way you will get passed! It's like getting chased by a bear! But as it turns out, that was not the case. As the only student left without a partner, I was tasked with keeping count of my own laps as I ran.

And this is where a new thought crept in: I was in control. I could control how many laps I ran. No one else was counting. If push came to shove, I could always change the number to avoid a little humiliation.

I was in control of the numbers.

As we lined up to get ready to go, some of my classmates started discussing strategy. Most agreed that we would all run a lap and then walk a lap. That sounded easy enough: one lap giving it my all and one lap to rest. Repeat. I could do that. I could keep it up.

The teacher said go and off we went. With my heart already racing from nerves, the first lap was much harder than I thought. Halfway through I was already out of breath. It was going to be hard for me to keep going, but I did. I didn't want to finish last on the first lap!

As our group finished the first lap I was instantly relieved. I could start my walking lap and catch my breath a little before we started to run again. As I slowed, I noticed that most of my other classmates didn't. They had abandoned our run/walk strategy right away and settled into a comfortable pace! What happened to our plan? That was not an option for me. My fear started to come true; I was last.

And on top of that, I was struggling. I could barely jog at this point, let alone run. At this point my goal was less about finishing the mile and more about staying alive. I had pain in every part of my abdomen. The crowd of students standing on the blacktop counting their partners' miles but their partners had a front row seat to my misery. I could feel them staring at me. I could sense their laughter. And it all felt like failure.

Eventually other runners began to catch up and lap me. I'd gone from being on my own to lost in the middle of the pack. There was a newfound sense of safety there; no one knew what lap I was on. For all they knew, I was running right with them, not a lap behind them. Eventually I had a friend catch up to me. I decided I would muster any energy I had and run with him. I asked him what lap he was on while he was passing me, and when he replied, "Eight," I quickly said, "Me too!"

As we passed a group of kids, they started cheering.

"Go Ben and... Jesse?"

They were completely shocked that I would be running right alongside Ben, and rightfully so. Ben was much more in shape, healthier, and skinnier than I was. He had all the things that would say to others he should be able to run the mile without stopping. He should be in front of Jesse, so how in the world was Jesse running with Ben?

The truth was that I wasn't. My actual lap count was probably half his at that point, but there was no way I was going to say it. Lap 8--that was my new count. And everyone watching was surprised and impressed that I was running with Ben. That's what I wanted. I wanted approval from my peers. For a second, it felt good.

As faster runners started to finish their mile, the crowd began to thin. As I looked around at the few of us left running, I reminded myself of my earlier resolve: I could not finish last. And even if it meant lying about my lap count, I was in control of that. So I made my way over to the coach and asked her my time.

11:58

I had just completed the mile run in 11:58. I remember that number like it was yesterday. For some reason that number has stayed with me as a constant reminder of my mile experience.
Except that I hadn't really completed the mile run, but I was the only one who knew that. And because no one else knew, I avoided the humiliation of being last. That was good enough for me.

Covering up the truth about that mile was exactly that: a cover up. I wanted to appear as something I was not, and this was just one way to do it. There's no real advantage to cheating or cutting corners. It only develops a false sense of security. But when that false sense of security fades, what are you left with?

Reality.

And after that day, my reality was the same: I was still the "big kid." Cheating on my mile time did not give me any sense of confidence. It didn't make me feel better about myself. I was still making choices that were unhealthy. I still wanted to change.

But how? I didn't know how. I assumed it was going to be like this forever. And that feeling is horrible. To assume you're always going to be a certain way is in a sense a way of giving up or giving in to the circumstances. By no means was that the truth. Sometimes it takes more than willpower to change. Sometimes it takes a team of people to help but I've learned that doing life with others and leaning on them for help is a great way to do life!

Mile

5

Plans

I like a plan. I like predictability. I like to think that if I follow a plan, I'll always know what's coming. It's a sense of control for me. I can predict the outcome.

I developed this habit of planning early in life. It started out innocent enough. With my parents' work schedules, I was often in charge of getting ready for school on my own before the bus arrived at 6:30 am. So I would plan ahead.

Every day I would get up, take a shower, and grab breakfast. My typical breakfast usually consisted of a Pop Tart, donuts, or something else premade and readily available in our pantry. If my parents were home they would cook pancakes (a specialty of my dad's) or egg sandwiches. After I ate I was out the door. I had to lay my clothes out the night before. If I didn't have any clothes laid out and ready to go, I would get a horrible night's sleep. I would toss and turn wondering what I had to wear. You wouldn't think this would be a concern for a young boy but for some reason, it mattered to me.

After school it was always snack time. My parents didn't get home until well after 5:00 every day so snack time was up to me. This is where my unhealthy decisions really started to affect my life. Chicken potpie, frozen sausage links, potato chips-- those were routine on my snack menu. Snack time was something that I looked forward to. You would think that an elementary school kid would look forward to coming home and playing with friends but not me. It was time to eat, and eat alone! There was no one else around and eating made me feel good.

Looking back now, I see my choices were never healthy. I began to overeat very young. It wasn't a matter of if I was hungry or not; I just made it part of my plans. My plans consisted of things that made me feel good, and food was high on that list. Plans can be a good thing but my planning was focused around mealtimes and food. Planning my food is something I thought I wanted-- something I thought I needed. I realize now that it wasn't the food I was looking forward to but the comfort and release it gave me from school, peers, and the pressure of trying to fit in. I would finally be able to decompress from school, and food helped allow me to do that. And I liked it. That's why I included food in my afternoon routine everyday.

This was a time when the subtle thoughts would encourage my unhealthy overeating. The thoughts would say things like, "See how good that tastes and makes you feel? You need more of those." That's how I developed bad and binging eating habits that were not healthy. It was all about how eating the food made me feel.

Food became my top priority when it came to plans. If I were going outside to play with friends, I would plan ahead and bring a snack just in case I got hungry. It didn't matter how long I would be gone or if I had just eaten. I had to factor food into my plans.

That after school snack time was a comfort to me. It was just me. No one saw me eating. I didn't feel the judgment of other people. I just ate. Even though I thought I was in control because I had plans, my plans focused around food and that gave me a false sense of security.

Now while there's certainly nothing wrong with an after school snack, there's definitely something wrong with the choices I was making.

By the time elementary school came to a close, I weighed approximately 170 pounds. That's not an extreme obese weight, but definitely one that made me the larger one of my group. My weight discouraged me. My weight made me think less of myself. I thought if I was skinnier, I would be normal.

Being in 6th grade and 170 pounds certainly wasn't part of the plan. I planned to stop being the "big kid." I planned to turn myself into the "normal kid." And while I really wanted to, I couldn't magically make it happen. I didn't really even know how to start.

These early years in my life built a foundation for what happened later in my life during my struggle with anorexia. As a kid I was consumed with food. I liked the way it made me feel and the comfort it gave me, but those were feelings that shouldn't come from food. They were leading me to eat when I wasn't hungry. They were leading me to eat for the wrong reasons.

For athletes, food can be a priority. And when it's focused on nutrition, hydration, and what your body needs to work at optimal potential, that's not necessarily a bad thing. My focus started with nutrition. I was hyper focused on what made my body work at it's best, but soon that would change. I can't tell you why I would eat during snack time when I wasn't hungry or why I would make the wrong food decisions as a kid. It's the same reason I can't tell you why I became obsessed with the scale instead of fueling my body. The best explanation I have is that it was built on the fear of becoming the kid I once was--the kid who had no control, no plan, and felt excluded from life because of being overweight. The thought of being lonely again and returning to outcast status was not pleasant. Thinking back on times when as the "big kid," I wondered what other people are saying about me wasn't fun. Those feelings and that season of life are things I didn't want to live again.

As an adult, some parents have asked me how they could help their child. What should they say? How should they respond to comments their child makes about their size, weight, or appearance? What helped me the most was trying to figure out why. Recovery is very hard and very ugly. It's a constant struggle between what you know you need to do and the irrational thinking that tells you that you shouldn't do it. Throughout my recovery when I would say things like, "I shouldn't eat that food," my wife wouldn't argue with me. She would simply ask, "Why do you feel like that?" She helped me focus on why I felt the way I did about food and talk through my thoughts. Starting with why is a good place to start.

Mile

6

Middle school

Reality check.

That's what they should call middle school: a three-year reality check.

Before I got to middle school, I assumed it would be just the same as elementary school. School is school, right?

That couldn't have been further from the truth.

For starters, I had gone from an elementary school whose total enrollment around 350 to a seventh grade class of close to 800. Talk about overwhelmed.

I quickly noticed that while I used to be one of the taller kids in class that was no longer the case. Kids I had seen just a few months ago were now almost as tall as my dad! And they were skinny, too! How was I going to shift attention from my weight when kids were sprouting up and thinning out left and right? My perception of myself continued to decline. The feelings were subtle, but they were still there--feelings of insecurity, embarrassment, and guilt. Of course Eddie was there, telling me it was all my fault. No one else was feeding me; I was doing it to myself.

And don't get me started on the wardrobe! In elementary school you could wear whatever you wanted. The coolest kid in class could wear a shirt filled with holes for days in a row, and no one would notice. But middle school--this was a different ball game! Kids were wearing collared shirts, dressing up, combing their hair, and generally putting effort into their appearance. The kids I knew in elementary school--their faces looked the same but everything else about them seemed totally different!

Needless to say, the first day of middle school didn't go as well as I'd hoped, and it all culminated in science class.

Science class started out just like any other. The teacher took attendance, went over the rules, and assigned seats for the semester. I was pleased with my seat--second from the back and right in front of my friend Alicia from elementary school.

I loved Alicia because of her laugh. It was the kind of laugh that just made your day better. And even better, she laughed at everything I said. While some would roll their eyes or ignore your jokes, Alicia would throw her head back and laugh.

Beside Alicia was Julie. She was new to me, a tall and athletic girl who seemed to be friendly. She went right to work friending Alicia. I listened to their conversation the first day as Julie made comments about her schedule, the activities she was going to do, and new people she had met. Their conversation sounded much more interesting than what the teacher was saying! Then came the comment that took me by surprise and will forever be etched in my brain.

"Alicia, how can you see the teacher with this big headed kid sitting in front of you?"

Wait a minute! Was she talking about me? No one had ever made fun of me like that before. At least not when they knew I could hear them! She was just joking. I mean, she couldn't have been serious. Maybe she has jokes, too!

But then came the next one. And the one after that. Julie's comments kept coming, and it was only the first day. She noticed what I hoped every other kid didn't: my size. She talked about how big I was constantly.

I couldn't see Alicia's expressions as it happened, but I could feel them. And that only added to my humiliation.

What did I do? Well, what any kid getting made fun of on their first day of middle school would do. I sat there and took it. I didn't say a word, and just pretended not to hear.

But I heard every word, and I carried them with me for years to come. Eddie used these words in a powerful way, both then and later during my battle with anorexia. He reminded me of those words, holding them over me as a reminder of what I would become if I were to eat and not run. If I ate normally and didn't run, I would surely gain weight. Who's to say the weight gain would stop? Would I stop caring about being skinny? Would it start a snowball of weight gain that I wouldn't be able to control?

That day in middle school, I believed Eddie was right. Everyone was older, but nothing had changed. It had been years since the humiliation of the mile run, and still the same things were happening. It made me think that maybe I should listen to Eddie a little more. Besides, he'd been right about pretty much everything up to this point. Maybe he could help me from here on out. At least that's what I thought.

Middle school continued much like that first day. Julie continued to make comments about my appearance. I continued to pretend I didn't hear them. The only thing that seemed worse to me than the comments themselves were people finding out that they actually hurt me.

As time went on, I started to notice that some of the other "big kids" in my class were losing weight. They seemed to be becoming stronger and more athletic, but I wasn't. I couldn't understand how it could happen for them, but not for me. I felt completely out of control. Being out of control isn't somewhere I like to be. Why couldn't I change like them? Eddie kept reminding me that I was always going to be the "big kid" so I had to find ways to adjust to that life.

Oddly enough I found solace in PE class. While I didn't look on the outside like a kid who would love athletic activity, I really did enjoy sports, and PE gave me a chance to show it. At least until the teacher mentioned the fitness test.

It was my worst nightmare all over again. As she listed every exercise required of us to complete the fitness test-- pull-ups, sit-ups, and of course, the elusive mile run--I was riddled with anxiety. I had saved myself the public humiliation of the mile run in elementary school, but I didn't see how I could do it now. So when the day came, I was more than a little worried.

The test would begin with pull-ups and sit-ups. All the students were asked to line up behind the pull-up bar. When your name was called, you were to jump onto the bar and do as many pull-ups as you could in the given timeframe.

While I hoped to be lucky enough to go after another student who might struggle, my name was called quickly, and so I was up to the bar. When the teacher said go, I tried as hard as I could to pull myself up on the bar, but gravity was not on my side. There was nothing I could do about it. I couldn't do a single pull-up. Because I was facing the wall, I was relieved not to be able to see the expressions of the other kids in class. I just wanted to get this over with as quickly as possible.

After what felt like an eternity hanging on the bar, the teacher called time, and I was back on the sidelines watching others take their turn. To my surprise, few comments were made about my failure on the pull-up bar. I laughed it off, but wondered what everyone else might be thinking. I had tried to convince people that perhaps my size didn't mean I was unhealthy; maybe it meant I was strong. But the pull-up test had just proved that wasn't true.

I didn't have time to dwell on that; up next was the mile run.

Obviously, I hadn't spent much time training for my next mile after the failed attempt in elementary school. But here I was again, and this time there was no cheating.

The PE coach stood at the lap checkpoint herself and made note on a paper of how many laps each student completed. There was no way to control the numbers this time. I knew it was going to be hard, but I went at it with one goal: not to embarrass myself. This time we were on a dirt track, and the mile consisted of only four laps around the track. I know the loop was just bigger, but hopefully the four laps would go by faster.

I lined up alongside my classmates and focused on the laps ahead. The whistle blew, and we were off! As we started, I found myself keeping pace with the other kids.

Maybe this time I can do it. Maybe this mile will go better than the last.

But we hadn't even made it halfway around the track before I found myself short of breath. I slowed to a walk just shy of completing one lap. I was surprised by how many others in my class were able to run without stopping for such long periods of time. I wanted so badly to run alongside them, but I had no idea how to get to that point. At the time, it genuinely felt impossible to me. That's a rough spot to be in as a kid. I'd go as far to say it's even tough as an adult. The feeling of impossibility can be very destructive on your confidence, and it was especially damaging to my self-confidence.

I continued to alternate between running and walking for the remainder of the mile. It felt like forever! I was so thankful for those classmates who chose to walk the entire mile. Thanks to them, I didn't come in last. Total embarrassment averted again!

While I didn't want to appear completely drained, I couldn't hide it. I had no energy left. Finishing the mile took everything I had, but I finished. I didn't have to cut any corners. I didn't have to fib any numbers. I completed it all on my own. That has to be something to celebrate, right? There was as small sense of accomplishment at the end of the mile. I mean, I finished a mile. At that age, it felt like a long way. I had a small sense of pride for what I had accomplished.

Nothing else mattered in middle school other than fitting in. Fitting in meant having friends, and that's what I wanted. But being the "big kid" made fitting in and having friends feel more difficult to me. My self-esteem was at an all time low. So to cover it up, I pulled away. I became increasingly introverted. If I kept to myself then others wouldn't notice me, right? If I don't let anyone in, I won't get hurt.

But I had run the mile. I had climbed Mt. Everest. It may have taken a sundial to time me, but I did it. It was over. And it brought a small sense of hope for what might be to come.

Practice Runs
The high from completing my first mile didn't last long. I knew the inevitable truth: eventually, I was going to have to do it again. The year was far from over and the PE coach had informed us early on that the fitness test would take place again at the end of the semester to gauge our improvements.

The next time wouldn't take me by surprise. This time I would come ready. I hadn't ever prepared for the mile before. I figured I'd give it a shot. Why not? What was there to lose? I was going to create and follow a plan in hopes of having a better outcome.

It was simple: I would practice running. Everyday after school I would run a little outside to see how far I could get. My family lived on eight acres of land so there was plenty of space. I just had to get to it. My obsessive tendencies kicked in. If I was going to do something I was going to put everything I had into it and do it the best I could.

So I grabbed my shoes, checked my stopwatch, and headed out for my first practice run.

It was just Eddie and me. I didn't know he was going to tag along, but he sure made his presence felt. The process of prepping for the run was tough enough, but Eddie made it tougher. He was constantly in my ear, saying things like, "You aren't getting any better," or "You know you're never going to be a runner. Stop wasting your time."

Nonetheless, I pushed on. Start at the line, start the watch, and just go for as long as I could.

Just like that I was off.

I followed the route toward my grandparents' house then down a hill and towards our pond. Up to this point running wasn't going that bad. By the time I made it to the pond, I was surprised to have some energy left. I kept going until I made it to the halfway point--the bench where my brother and I would sit to fish--before I needed to stop.

I was out of breath, and my muscles were screaming. It felt like something had stabbed me in the side of my chest. My lungs were burning, but I had made it that far. And so I started again, this time moving back up the hill. Much harder. Much more painful.

As I crossed the imaginary finish line to the front steps of my house, I turned and looked back at my route. I wasn't sure how far I had run--maybe half of a mile? In all honesty, the distance didn't matter much. I ran on my own. I made it back in one piece. This was the first step to help me get to where I wanted to go. It wasn't a first step to the physical goal of finishing a mile; it was the first step to understanding that I could do really good things when I set my mind on a goal, worked hard, and didn't give up.

The path to bettering yourself is never easy. In order to get better at anything, it takes hard work, dedication, a plan, others to encourage you, and, from my experience, patience. Improvement takes times. It won't happen overnight--especially with running. You'll see the benefits from running only after putting in a dedicated amount of time and work.

So I continued. The next day as I headed out for my second practice run, I felt different. Any runner will tell you that there's always a little bit of anxiety that hits you prior to a run. No matter how long you've been doing it, the questions creep in: Can I make it that far? Am I going to hit my goal? But that day, I felt no such thing. Was I an athlete now? I had completed a run the day before and that was a huge   deal   for   me.

Standing before my second practice run, I didn't feel any trace of anxiety. I felt full of possibility. Today was another opportunity to better myself. Who would have thought even just a few weeks ago I would be following a plan to run a mile?

With the final fitness test just a few weeks away, I continued my practice runs two to three times a week. Our final grade was dependent on improving--no matter how little--from our first test. Failure just wasn't an option.

One day as I was preparing for one of my afternoon runs, I breezed past my mom and tossed out an invitation to join me. Much to my surprise, she answered, "Sure!" There had not been one day in my entire life that I'd seen my mom run other than from the car to the house in the rain. Being a parent now I can attest to the fact that when you see your kids doing something that will better their lives, you will do anything in your power to encourage them to keep going. I believe this was the case with my mom that day.

I had yet to run with anyone else, and I found myself wondering how I would do now running alongside a partner. I laid out the route for her before we started, and then we took off together. I tracked with her for a bit, towards my grandparents' house and down the hill--the common weekly route by now. By the time I passed the bench I noticed she was no longer with me. I couldn't see or hear my mom anywhere nearby. I stopped to look back and saw she had slowed to a walk pretty far behind me.

And it hit me: I wasn't last. I had actually run longer and faster than someone else, and I had some energy left to keep going! Even if she was in front of me I could still tell myself I was in second place.. of two runners.

I continued on and made it the entire lap without stopping. After taking a short break, I was back to running again. This was by far the longest I had run without giving in before, and I wasn't about to quit now. As I finished my second lap I saw my mom again, not too far in front of me. And a new thought occurred: could I catch her? Maybe even pass her?

There's a lot to be said for not finishing last, but more about actually passing someone. That would be incredible. I had never in my life been in the position to pass anyone in any kind of endurance challenge.

As I approached my third lap, I did it. I not only caught up to my mom, but I actually passed her. It was exhilarating. I officially hit my first "runner's high." Before running just hurt, but now I was beginning to get some strange satisfaction from running. Don't get me wrong, it still hurt, but now there was something to be proud of with the pain.
I completed three laps and beat my mom. Did it matter that her age exceeded mine by decades? No. Did it matter that she probably saw me coming and slowed her pace to a crawl as I approached? Not one bit. What mattered was that I had done it. In just three laps, I had done more than I ever thought I could do.

Something started to happen inside my spirit over the next few weeks. I actually started to enjoy running. I liked the challenge. I would test myself differently each time, sometimes with distance and sometimes with speed. It certainly wasn't easy. There were days when I felt like my family might find me passed out in the woods from an excruciatingly difficult run. But I was still running.

And then the day finally came: I ran one entire mile without stopping. I didn't have it completed measured. I don't know if it was an actual mile, but the loop around my pond seemed pretty close to the loop around the football field. But I didn't stop there. I kept going another lap after that. Sure it was only a little over a mile, but to me, it might as well have been a marathon. I couldn't believe it.

With the second fitness test just days away, I knew I would be ready.

The Third Mile

To say I was focused on the next fitness test would be an understatement. As the day approached, it consumed my every thought. Could I actually do it? Would this practice pay off? I kept trying to tell myself that no matter what happened, it wouldn't be worse than the time before. Somehow that still didn't calm my nerves.

And then the day came.

Together, our class made its way down to the dirt track. We stretched a little and made our way to the line. Our teacher explained the process again, but this time the stakes were higher. The faster you ran, the higher your grade. In order to get an A, your run had to come in under an eight-minute mile. If I could just get a C, that would be enough! And just as with the miles before, my primary goal remained the same: don't embarrass yourself.

Once again, we were off! I paced myself at the start of our run, hoping to just run two laps before needing to take a break. As I rounded the first lap, the coach shouted out my time: "1:56." And then the second lap: "3:58." She seemed just as surprised as I was to tell me I'd run the first half-mile in under four minutes. Somehow I was on track to get an A!

At this point I should tell you that I'm a South Carolina Gamecock fan. We are used to playing good for one half, taking satisfaction that we kept it close, and then getting outplayed considerably in the second half. This was my expectation for the final two laps of my race that day, but I figured I'd give it a shot!

Hearing my time was the motivation I needed and so I pushed on, continuing to run throughout the third lap. I began to notice that I was running alongside other kids who were much faster than me during the last test. We were all on the same lap, and I was keeping up! This reality pushed me on to keep running and finish the third lap.

I was in pain. My side was splitting. My feet felt like they were in quicksand. The teacher shouted out my time again: "Jesse Harmon 5:57." These numbers are still ingrained in my mind and probably forever will be. The numbers calculated success for me. It communicated how my hard work had paid off. I'll never forget the teacher's expression as she called out my times. It was an incredible experience.

I couldn't believe I'd made it this far in six minutes. I had definitely already hit my goal to avoid embarrassment and that could have been enough. But for some reason, this time, it wasn't.

The reality hit me that if I just kept running this final lap at the same speed I could actually finish this mile in less than eight minutes and earn my A. I had a chance!

Even though I was moving a little slower and struggling to breathe, I didn't stop. I gave it my all. My chest was pounding, and I was in pain. I tried to come up with hand signals to tell my PE coach that I needed an ambulance, but I couldn't figure out how to communicate my need non-verbally. I didn't know if anyone had died doing the mile run before but I surely felt I would be the one.

And as I approached the line, I knew that no matter if I got that A or not, I had achieved something I never thought possible. I had run an entire mile without stopping. In front of everyone, I didn't quit. I was an athlete, and everyone saw it.

I think my teacher was more excited than I was as I crossed the finish line. She had no idea the work I had put in behind the scenes, but she saw the improvement. She shouted excitedly: "Jesse Harmon 7:56!"

I ran a mile. I got an A. I felt like an athlete. I proved to Julie and everyone else who I really was inside. I hoped everyone saw it, heard it, or read it. It's a feeling I wish on everyone. I completed something that I thought would never be possible. I completed a mile in less than eight minutes. To me, that was Olympic standard. At the time, it gave me hope that I could be something and do something with my life. Up to that point, I believed it wasn't a possibility because of the limitations that came with being the "big kid." But what I learned that day is that potential is readily available to anyone of any size, shape, or color. Potential is out there for anyone's taking. Running was teaching me how to pursue my potential. And I realized that the same values I was learning through preparing for the mile--hard work, dedication, and patience--were the same that could help me reach other goals in my life.

That mile was such a proud moment in my life. And another added bonus? It shut Eddie up for awhile!

Note: While I was in counseling, I was able to identify how my experiences as a youth influenced food decisions I made while battling anorexia. I didn't realize in middle school that the impressions and tendencies I was developing were that of an eating disorder. I learned this in counseling with the help of a licensed professional. I strongly encourage someone who wants to fully recover to discuss a plan with a licensed professional.

Mile

7

Words

Words are powerful to me. They're affirming. They're life giving. They're the way I receive love. If you want to let me know how you feel about me, I want you to put it into words.

I think I developed this affinity for words in middle school. I learned the hard way how powerful a word spoken could be.

"There is one whose rash words are like sword thrusts, but the tongue of the wise brings healing." (Proverbs 12:18)

Words can be deadly. It's scary to think how quickly words come out of our mouths before we give them much thought. They can do irreparable damage when we use them that way. I've always been able to remember the negative things people say to me for a long time. Sometimes I use them as motivation, but no matter what, it's hard to brush them off. I wish it were easier for me to deal with people's verbal opinions, but it's a continual struggle. I think that's one reason why middle school was so damaging to me on a personal level. Granted, any middle school kid will say things they don't mean or think are harmless. Those words just stuck with me longer than middle school.

The negative words from middle school fueled Eddie's pressure when I was battling anorexia. There were countless times he would rekindle feelings of loneliness and seclusion I felt because of my weight. He would say things like, "You don't want to be that again. You want to run more in order to stay thin," or "You ate too much today. You need to go burn off a few more calories."

Negative words from my childhood built within me a fear of not wanting to be the "big kid" again. They motivated my goal to make sure I did not become the kid I once was.

"Whoever guards his mouth preserves his life; he who opens wide his lips comes to ruin." (Proverbs 13:3)

Middle school is hard on everyone. That's just the truth. No matter how cool you think you are, middle school will tell you otherwise. It felt like the deck was stacked against me back then. I physically changed, but much slower than other guys. I didn't grow four inches taller when they did. I didn't develop obvious muscle tone like they did. I remained overweight, younger than most kids in my class, and physically maturing much slower than the rest. Needless to say, fitting in was hard.

So I began a new course of action. I wasn't obsessed with having a million friends. I didn't have to fit in. I just wanted people to say good things about me. I wanted their words to be positive. That would be enough.

But there was still Julie. I believe every middle school has a Julie. She's the person who takes pleasure in pointing out your every fault, mishap, and imperfection. Nothing gets passed her--at least nothing that would humiliate someone else.

I still remember to this day some of the words she used in pointing out the supposed flaws she saw in me. Words like "fat," "smells bad," and "needs to lose some weight." She made every day in seventh grade science class a miserable experience. She branded those words into my brain over the course of the semester, and as hard as I tried to forget them, I couldn't.

She didn't know the power of her words. At least I hope she didn't. For me, her words made me question the most important thing about myself, my value. They made me feel worthless. But there was still a sense of fight in me. I still had the willpower to want to change. There was a motivating factor in her negative words. I knew I wanted to change, and I was going to do it. I was going to try to make myself different.

Mile

8

Church

It was the summer before my sophomore year (Freshman year was still at the middle school). Middle school was finally behind me, and the freedom of high school was on the horizon.

Like most kids, summers for me consisted of playing outside, swimming, and staying up later than usual, free from the time constraints of school. It also included weekends with my grandparents.

And weekends with my grandparents meant going to church.

Church wasn't a huge part of my family's life. My parents never made it a priority to go. It didn't seem like it mattered much to them, and I figured that if it didn't matter much to them, then it probably wasn't that important. My grandparents certainly thought church was important so if we were staying with them on a Sunday morning, we were going to church.

So one Sunday during the summer before high school, I loaded up and went to church with my grandparents. I had been there before and knew what to expect: an hour in Sunday school, an hour in the main service, and then home. That day at church started as most other trips to church did; we went to our designated class and waited for Sunday school to start. But then something new and different happened. I actually recognized someone from school--a friend. I had no idea that I knew anyone who went to this church--let alone someone I would actually be glad to see. Then the next thing I knew, another kid I recognized walked in. And then another. I was surprised to see them just as much as they were surprised to see me. This church thing was shaping up to actually be fun!

I wish I could tell you that it was because of a great lesson from my Sunday School teacher or an incredible sermon from the preacher, but for a 15-year-old kid, it was all about friends, and I really wanted friends. With friends found at church, I decided I would go back. The feeling of being accepted by a group of my peers was great. It was exactly what I needed at the time.

Those first few weeks going to church were a little awkward for me. I didn't grow up in church so while other kids could answer every question in Sunday school and find every book in the Bible without a problem, I had no clue. But what I loved about church was that even though I didn't really fit in with the kids there, no one ever made a point to let me know. No one acted like I was different. One thing was for sure: there was a lot more grace at church than there was at school.

Time came to register for church summer camp, and I found myself actually wanting to go. That's saying a lot for a kid who had never stayed multiple nights away from his parents--let alone out in the woods at camp! But if my newfound friends were going, I was in!

Camp that summer was exactly how you would imagine it to be. Cabins in the woods, a huge pond for swimming, activities to do outside all day long--it was incredible. The days at camp were spent with friends and fun, but the nights were turned over to a guest speaker. He shared with us things about God that I had never heard before. His message was simple: God had created us each uniquely. God had given each of our lives a purpose. God could use each of us for His good.

I was sure he couldn't be talking about me. I mean, how in the world could He use a guy like me to do anything? I could barely run the mile, remember? I didn't think my life had the potential to have any sort of purpose so the fact that with God it did was a message I had never heard before. And I was intrigued. It was like drinking water out of a fire hydrant. I wanted to decide if what this guy was saying was actually true. Could I really have a purpose? Could I really make a difference? Why does this God find value in me? All of these thoughts were going through my mind as I listened. I was a teenager trying to grasp the answers to these major questions. It seemed like a routine message to others based on their expressions, but for me, it was all new.

I had been listening to others to determine my value. I had let the numbers determine my value. I was overweight, I was slow, and the numbers on the scale proved that I wasn't normal.

The idea that I had value to God changed everything for me. And so on Wednesday, June 23rd, I decided to join God's team.

I had been in church services before where music was played and everyone would wait to see if anyone was going to get up and talk to the preacher about giving their lives to God. But this time was different. I wanted to be that guy that got up. I wanted to give my life to God. I decided to believe that I had value and purpose. I wanted to do something with my life. I knew God loved me, died for me, and because of that I wanted to make an impact for Him.

So I got up. I walked to the front, and I tried to pray. I'd never really prayed before that moment so what came out was a little jumbled. I asked God to forgive me for the things I might have done wrong along the way. I prayed that He would help me understand my purpose so that I might help others do the same. And just like that, I was on His team.

It felt incredible. I actually felt different. It was like a release of pressure--like letting out a breath I didn't even know I was holding. There was a newfound power in knowing that God designed me. I had a purpose. God loved me.

And to Him, I was valuable.

That value was communicated through the friends I made at church. Church was great for me. It helped me understand that I was created for so much more than I thought and believed. I met Christian friends at the height of need in my life and had a great team of adults that wanted to help me no matter what. I'm reminded often that it takes caring adults to help young people understand they have potential and can do something with their lives. Unfortunately, the feeling of purpose doesn't come naturally. I wish all young people understood that they have incredible amounts of potential and purpose, but unfortunately it usually doesn't happen until someone comes alongside them and helps them see it.

I mention church in my story because my faith was foundational for me during my healing process. Throughout recovery there were many times it was just me. I was alone and trying to get better. The process to recovery is tough and painful and during times of prayer, God reminded me of my value and purpose. Someone once told me that as long as I still have air in my lungs, I have tangible, living proof that God still has a purpose for my life.

Even after becoming a Christian, Eddie would still visit from time to time. He was always there. There was always a fear of being overweight again. I promised myself I would never be that kid I was in elementary school. For Christmas my junior year of high school I asked for a weight machine. I had learned from my experience training for the mile that hard work can pay off, and so my plan was to use the machine to help keep me from being the fat kid again.

Watching the movie *The Hurricane* was a defining moment for me as a teenager as well. It was a true story of Ruben "Hurricane" Carter who had been jailed and suspected of killing innocent people. One part from the movie is still branded into my brain. While in his jail cell Ruben said he would not conform to the system because he knew he was innocent, but instead he turned his body into a machine. He would do sit-ups in his jail cell. He made sure his body could operate at optimal potential.

When I heard that, I knew that's what I wanted. I wanted to be stronger and faster than any other person. I wanted to turn my body into a machine. I wanted no person to have the opportunity to make fun of me or point out any of my insufficiencies. I was still the slow kid from Red Bank. There was no way I was going to be the fastest or strongest, but I was motivated to try.

And of course, Eddie was there to cheer me on, twisting and affirming every thought. He was constantly whispering for me to work harder. Just like he used food to make me feel good and give me identity, he was now using exercise to do the same. He used the fear of being the "big kid" to motivate me to work out harder. Now while there's nothing wrong with working out and lifting weights, it's certainly not healthy when motivated by fear. And fear was my primary motivator to exercise.

It ignited a training regime that I kept through the remaining years in high school. I would work out and try to stay in shape. I would always stay very aware of how my body looked. I made sure I wasn't gaining weight and avoid clothes that made me look heavy. I'm sure this sounds odd coming from a guy, but my fear kept me aware of my appearance. I was hesitant to eat certain foods because I wanted to be skinny.

Soon, I developed the habit of avoiding school lunch. I remember wondering how other kids at school could eat a slice of pizza everyday for lunch and not be overweight? Instead of eating lunch I opted for a soda and a roll of chewy candy from the vending machine. Of course now I know that from a nutrition perspective my food choices were much worse than those offered at school lunch, but at the time I didn't know any different. I thought less food meant a better outcome.

My poor food decisions continued through college. I went to North Greenville University for my the first two years, and I remember multiple days where I would eat a bagel for breakfast, a bagel for lunch and a bagel for dinner. Why? I was afraid of gaining weight. I was all too aware of the potential for the infamous freshman 15. I didn't want to become one of those college students who gained that weight their freshman year. I didn't want to be fat.

Those years were full of disordered eating habits. I wasn't eating enough, and I wasn't eating the right things. I had a distorted perception of food and what it would do to my body. I believed food would make me gain weight, and in my eyes, there was no fate worse than that.

Mile

My first race

College life is fun. You meet new friends from all over the country. It's almost like hitting a reset button on your life. Most of the time no one has a clue who you are or what your story is. The things that seemed to matter so much in high school just don't matter as much anymore. It's almost like summer camp (except for the eventual homework).

My first weeks as a student at North Greenville College were exciting, hanging out with new friends and meeting new people. One day in the cafeteria I met some students who were on the cross-country team. They shared stories of preparing for an upcoming race, and, while I wished them luck, I knew in my mind there was no way I would ever want to run a race. But every time I saw them running around campus, something looked different about them. They actually looked like they *enjoyed* running.

It made me think back to my fitness test in middle school and all those practice runs. While I never enjoyed them, I did feel a sense of accomplishment after each one. And the thought entered my mind: maybe I could actually enjoy running. Maybe I should give it a try.

So I laced up my shoes and started going for runs around campus. And something surprising happened: I actually *wanted* to keep going. I don't know if it was because I enjoyed the runs or just the thought that I might be impressing the girls on campus, but either way, I kept on going.

Running slowly became a hobby. I would scour the Internet, researching what shoes to wear, how to train, what types of food I should eat. I wanted to know as much as I could about this new, burgeoning passion.

Mile

10

Love

I met Sarah after my freshmen year of college. I was asked to speak at her church for a Sunday event celebrating graduating seniors. Since turning my life over to God I had become active in the local church and even found a little confidence as a speaker. It was easy to talk in front of people when I was talking about what God was doing in my life.

Just before I got up to speak, I noticed a little blonde girl standing up front, her head bobbing along with the music. I noticed how she sang along in the worship service and was impressed with how engaged she was in what was happening at church. And she was pretty easy on the eyes as well! Later, I eavesdropped as she talked to the person next to me about her recent breakup with her boyfriend. Bingo--I had a shot!

It took a little detective work on my part to learn more about her and a lot of guts to eventually ask her out. I wouldn't recommend my method to anyone because it's not how a guy should show his affection for a lady, but I chose to make my ask on AOL Instant Messenger. Now, while this incredible tool doesn't exist anymore, but in the words of Mr. T, I pity the fool that tries to ask my daughter out on a date via text message. Any future suitors better pick up the phone--just like I should have years ago! But nonetheless, Sarah agreed to the date.

Over the next four years, Sarah and I dated. Together we had opportunities to lead mission trips, volunteer with our youth group, and grow together in our relationship with each other but also with God. That was the most important thing to us. He was the foundation of our relationship, and He's what made it work.

One thing I loved about Sarah then (and still do today!) is what an encouragement she is to others around her. Her words speak life--and that's valuable to me! Her love for God and her willingness to serve other people for Him were the things that attracted me to her the most!

By my junior year of college I had transferred to Columbia International University to study youth ministry. It made such an impact on my life as a kid that I wanted to be a part of hopefully making that same impact on other kids in the future. Sarah studied at nearby Columbia College, pursuing a career as an elementary school teacher. After four years, as we approached our respective graduation dates, I knew it was time to take the next step.

So in January 2005, I dropped down on one knee and asked her to be my wife. Much to my delight (and relief!), she said yes. We were married the next summer in front of our family and friends. It was the best day, and there have been just a few days in my life that have even come close to it since.

At the time of our marriage I was healthy, weighing in at 185 pounds. Running was something I enjoyed as a hobby. I was also lifting weights during the week with the local high school football team. All of this felt like a balanced and healthy part of life.

To have someone like Sarah, who loved God and loved me, commit to spending the rest of her life with me was incredible. She agreed to stick with me for the long haul. She saw my value not in being a runner or an athlete or any of the things I'd thought had given me value up until that point; she saw my value in God. And I was so excited to start my life with her!

Today, as I think back on the vows we said that day, one part stands out more than any other: *in sickness and in health.* We vowed that to each other that day with no idea how true those words would soon become in our lives.

Mile

11

My second race

Soon after we took our vows I developed a training plan for my next 5k. I started in July 2006, just one month after Sarah and I got married. I wanted to know how to train so that I could improve as a runner. I read articles and found information online about race training and began to follow the instructions--even if they didn't make sense.

Being a planner, I wanted to set a goal. This time I would try to run the 5k in 21 minutes, setting my pace at a seven-minute mile.

I had a goal. I had a plan. Now it was time to start training. This race for me was different. Running was now different. I *wanted* to work hard. I *wanted* to set a goal and see if it was attainable. And so the date was set: September 3rd. I had half of July, all of August, and then the race. Not long to prepare, but long enough for me.

With my new time goal set, I started training. Each day I tried to run a mile in under seven minutes. To average a seven-minute mile for three miles straight was something I never thought possible for me, but I was motivated to see if it could be now. And I knew in order to try, I had to change more than just my running habits.

I began changing the way I ate to better accommodate my runs. I was like a walking science experiment, basing my decisions on what to eat on how my body responded during a run. It wasn't that I was suddenly started making healthier choices; I was just paying attention. Fried chicken fingers weren't as good for my runs as grilled chicken, and so I started swapping them out. For me, it was as simple as that: if it made me run better, I would eat it. Now just to be clear, there were a few non-negotiables for me when it came to food, for example, sweet tea. There was no way this Southern boy was giving up sweet tea!

With race day fast approaching, the urge to cram in workouts hit me hard. I did a lot of last minute runs. And as race day arrived, I wondered if it was enough to hit my goal.

Sarah showed full support leading up to the race. We had been married just three months and much of my time was occupied with this new training program. But as an encourager, Sarah was constantly supporting me as I worked hard to hit my goal (even if it meant doing a ton of extra laundry to keep all my workout clothes clean).

In a show of continued support, Sarah came with me to the race. The crowd was intimidating, full of what looked like real runners--tall, skinny athletes. But as nervous as I was about running against them, I was even more nervous about running against myself. In the past, my goal in a run was simply to finish, but this time my goal was to finish within a specific time, to beat the clock. I had made peace with the fact that I wasn't going to win the race overall, but I wanted to win it against my goal. I wanted to break that 21-minute time.

As the race director called everyone to the start line, I gave Sarah one last look and took my place. And just like that-the horn blew and we were off!

The course was an out and back, with runners going about a mile and a half before turning around to follow the same course in reverse to finish. With the first part of the race mostly downhill, I mentally prepared for the second part of the race to be a literal uphill battle. As I approached the turn around to lead me into the last mile and a half, I checked my watch. I was on track with my time, but it was close. I was going to have to keep working hard to hit my goal.

As I topped the hill, I caught site of the finish line, and gave it all I had. No matter what the race is, I've found that there's always a little extra boost that comes as I get close to the finish line. Maybe it's the crowd support. Or maybe it just knows the end is in sight. Either way, the boost helps get me over the line.

And that day was no exception. I rode the boost in energy all the way across the finish line and there was my time: 20.48. I'd done it. I hit my goal!

Sarah ran over to me and offered her congratulations. And then she said something I'll never forget: "I'm so proud of you!" In that moment, those words replaced everything that everyone else had said to me. They didn't matter anymore. I was a runner, and the person who mattered most was proud of it. And so was I.

As we drove home that day, I thought of the road I'd traveled with running. I had come so far in a relatively short time. I wasn't the person I used to be. I used to be so intimidated by running, but now I had voluntarily signed up for a three-mile road race. I actually paid money to run! Talk about change!

What happened that day was something I never thought possible. I didn't know I had it in me. I wasn't born with the gift of running. It didn't come easy for me. But I had worked hard. And that 5k showed me how hard work really can pay off. Finishing the race helped to silence the doubters. It helped to relieve the pressure of life. There was no pressure once I finished a run or a race, and that felt good. It was a feeling that I liked.

Mile

12

Keep running

After the race, my obsessive tendencies began to take over. I'm a very motivated person, and I set high goals for myself. I do as much as I can to reach my goals, and that's not always a bad thing. However, being obsessive about something can impact your life in a negative way. And that's the road I was headed down.

I started to pay close attention to my weight, my food, and my training. I cut fried foods from my diet. I didn't drink sugary carbonated drinks. In a few short months, I had lost between 15 and 20 pounds. I don't have a very large frame so the weight loss was pretty noticeable. I didn't see the weight loss as alarming though. I saw it as a result of hard work, and so I kept running and learning more about my passion.

My training runs looked a little different as I continued to run. I learned the value of pacing. I learned that if I started too fast then I wasn't going to be able to hold that pace to finish. And I learned how time really worked. I couldn't run a seven-minute mile for six miles straight, but I could still pace myself along the route to hit a 45-minute goal for a 10k run.

By October of 2006, I had run both a 5k and 10k. I felt free and felt confidence and I wanted more. I wanted to test the limits of my endurance. And so I signed up for a marathon. Yes, a 26.2-mile marathon (that's the only kind of marathon but sometimes it gets easily confused with other distances). I knew I needed time to train and that it would be difficult, but I was going to do it. The only thing left to do was find my next race--my marathon.

I found a race, I trained as hard as I knew how and I completed that first marathon in March 2007 with a time of 3:31:48. I narrowly missed my pace goal of eight minutes per mile. As I toed the line for the marathon, I had now lost 20 pounds, but again, that wasn't unusual for a first time marathon runner. My health felt better, and I loved my new found passion. I love endurance sports and how they made me feel. It gave me a sense of confidence. I was in control of how well I did and how fit I could become. Running quickly became a way for me to nurse my competitive spirit. I felt like I had something to prove to everyone. I had never been the runner, endurance athlete, or anyone's example of fitness, but now I wanted to be. It was up to me.

As I crossed the finish line of my first marathon, I felt proud of myself. I actually completed a marathon. I remembered all the negative things that were said about me in middle school. I remembered the seclusion. I remembered all the times I was made fun of in my youth. None of that could come close to exceeding the feeling of joy that came with completing that first marathon. It was exhilarating, and I was hooked.

Mile

13

The fade

The next three years brought a slow progression of weight loss. I was constantly cutting foods and working to get faster. I felt like I had discovered the formula I needed to become a successful endurance athlete. I just had to watch what I ate and consistently run.

Slowly, I began to cut more foods from my diet. I no longer drank sweet tea; it was only water. I didn't eat any desserts, fried foods, or soft drinks. I made sure to get plenty of carbs because I knew that carbs were fuel for a runner. A staple breakfast was two packets of instant oatmeal followed by three bowls of cereal, probably consuming around 200g of carbs for breakfast. It may seem like a lot, but it always left me energized and ready for a run after breakfast, but also a little guilt. Eddie would make sure I "knew" I had to run now. I couldn't eat that much food and not run, that's what he would tell me.

That was my typical routine: breakfast and then a run. Sometimes those runs would feel forced--like I didn't really want to do them. And to make matters worse, they were motivated by guilt because of how much I ate for breakfast. I was afraid of what would happen to my weight if I didn't run. And just like that, the passion for running was slowly being overtaken by the fear of gaining weight.

I started to hear Eddie's voice more around that time. Even if I wasn't hungry or didn't plan on running, I would consume the same amount of breakfast because I liked the way it tasted. And every time I would hear Eddie speak the same fears into my head about weight gain. He reminded me of my experiences as a kid. He made me feel guilty about what I ate. He made me beat myself up over my lack of self-control. Eddie was slowly convincing me that I was out of control, and the only way to take back control was to eat less or run more. But my running was going great. I was getting faster and running longer. So I had to be doing something right, right?

That's the one thing I've learned about Eddie now that I didn't realize then: he's a liar. Nothing he says is true, and there's no good reason to listen to him. His goal is to manipulate and destroy. I wasn't doing things right but the only way I knew to quiet his voice was to run.

I continued to lose weight and run. While I still had a passion for running, my fear of gaining weight was now gaining ground. In 2007 after my first marathon, I'd say I was only ten percent concerned with gaining weight, but as I approached 2009, that percentage was closer to fifty. Running released me from the guilt of what I ate. It started as a subtle thought, but soon, it became all about calculations for me. Most of my training, at the time, was done on a treadmill at the gym. I would weigh both before and after a run. Eventually, I knew how much I needed to run to reach a certain weight goal.

This fear began to grow when I made the decision to bike across the country. Approximately two years before my diagnosis, two friends and I rode from San Francisco to Yorktown, Virginia--more than 3,000 miles--to raise awareness for Crossover Athletics, a non-profit youth sports organization I oversee. I had no clue how difficult the ride would be or even how to train for it, but my friend Tony, who rode a lot, suggested we try to gain some weight prior to the trip to prepare for what we'd lose on the ride.

Before we left for the trip, I weighed around 153 pounds. I was nervous about the trip, not because of the physical challenge, but because I wouldn't be able to run. I hadn't taken a break from running in four years, and now I wouldn't be running for more than a month. Not running for me meant a possible weight gain and that scared me. Eddie had convinced me if I didn't run I would gain weight. If I gained weight then I would lose my fitness and my identity that was formed with running.

Now, if you're thinking that what I just said doesn't make any sense at all, you're absolutely right. Here I was about to bike across the country, and I was worried about not running! Eddie was feeding fear into my mind and with him, nothing was logical. He made me afraid that even on a 3,000-mile bike trip, I would somehow gain weight without being able to run.

Because of that, I became obsessed with the scale (yes, I brought a scale with me). I would weigh secretly everyday because I was embarrassed at the thought that my companions would see me. I let my weight during that trip control how much I ate each night. I didn't care about calories or even how I felt; the number on the scale determined everything. We were biking close to 100 miles a day, so there was no way I would be gaining weight.

Eddie became a part of my plans and when the other riders eventually saw me weighing in each day, I brushed it off as a deal I made with my wife to watch my health going across country. Of course that wasn't true. This deal I made with myself--with Eddie. I had to know the number to stay in control.

That was the first time I lied about my condition. Looking back, I see it as the starting point for the downward spiral of my disease. I was obsessed with my weight. I focused more on the scale than anything else. If I weighed in at night and I didn't like the number, I simply wouldn't eat much dinner to compensate. It didn't matter that I'd ridden for more than six hours that day. I was driven by fear, and it was slowly taking over my life.

During that trip I also started to reduce the amount of calories I was taking in overall. It was a choice fueled by fear and became almost like a challenge for me. I wanted to see if I could eat less than I did the day before. I wanted to see if I could control my tendency to overeat. I was hyper focused on food in a new way.

Each day brought a new challenge, and surprisingly none had to do with the actual ride. I was fearful of gaining weight. I couldn't run and didn't know how many miles I needed to ride to lose weight. I was miserable. It felt like a prisoner of sorts. I was prisoner to my own thoughts. I was completely helpless. I didn't want to think about food and the scale all the time, but, for the most part, I did.

The first thing I did when I arrived home was return to the gym to weigh in on what I thought was a better scale. Before the trip, my routine at the gym involved taking off my shoes and weighing in after I stretched. I did this before every workout, using the weight to determine how hard my workout needed to be. I needed to get back to this routine and see the number to know what I needed to do next. Before I weighed in I was nervous. The thought of weighing in was all I thought about. I knew I had gained weight. Was I going to be able to lose it? Was it the first pound back to becoming who I was? Those were the irrational thoughts that Eddie was sending me.

144.

When the number displayed on the scale, I was relieved. I hadn't gained weight. In fact, I'd actually lost weight. It was an odd and heavy weight off my shoulders (and my body!).

I felt in control. I had avoided a downward spiral into the person I used to be. And I thought if I could keep losing weight when I wanted to, I could somehow quiet Eddie's voice in my head. I could reassure him (and me) that I was in control. That number that day proved that I was in control.

But with every new number came a new routine from Eddie. He rejoiced with me as I saw that lower number on the scale. He whispered encouragement: "See, It's all about restriction. Just restrict a little of your diet and you can lose weight." He convinced me I was doing it right.

I created my own formula that let me know how many calories I would burn by running certain roads and areas around my house. My routine was, I weighed first thing in the morning, ate breakfast, and then weighed again. I wanted to drink water but I knew that liquid would add more weight so I only drank water as needed. After my breakfast weigh in, I would shower and then promptly weigh again. By the time I left the house for work, I would have weighed myself anywhere from four to six times. Yes, it was as miserable as it sounds.

My only relief would be to see that I had lost weight somewhere along the day, but that relief was only temporary. Every new weight brought a new fear of gaining even an ounce of it back. I stressed and worried over it all the time. Eddie convinced me that even one pound was the difference between control and lack of it.

The truth was that I needed to gain weight. I was incredibly unhealthy and mentally I had shifted. No longer was I worried about nutrition. I was solely focused on my weight numbers.

I was in the midst of a constant struggle between running and nutrition. I wasn't properly fueling my body, but my running times were still decreasing. Somehow I was getting faster. I had some close friends at that time mention how skinny I looked, but I couldn't convince myself it was unhealthy. I was a runner, and runners are skinny, right?

Deep down I knew my unhealthy habits were slowly destroying my body. I was binge eating--mostly at breakfast and on desserts. My running allowed me to eat in excess without having to reap the results of overeating on the scale. I didn't overeat often, but when I did I felt sick with guilt. I'm not talking about the occasional family reunion, stretchy pants type full, but the sick, drunken, type of full that comes from a combination of eating too much and guilt.

For example, during Thanksgiving leading up to one of my marathons, I went to my grandparent's house to eat lunch with my family. I knew I was going to overeat so I prepared for it by running ten-miles that morning. I was heavy into marathon training so I knew I could run off whatever I ate. I remember my Thanksgivings morning run vividly because I dreaded every step. I knew I wouldn't have any way to control my calorie intake at my grandparents so I had to get into a calorie deficit before I went. I calculated that I'd be down about 900 calories if I completed that run as planned. So with no energy and dragging my feet the whole way, I completed the run so I could eat lunch.

We went to lunch, and everything happened just as I suspected. I had no control over the amount of sweets I ate. I remember eating seven slices of chocolate cake. Now, while Nana's cake is good, it's not seven slices at once good! On the way home, I was frustrated with myself for the choice. My wife saw my frustration and tried to start a conversation about it, but I blew her off. All I could hear was Eddie. He kept saying, "You need to run. You need to run."

Eddie's voice was never about nutrition or health. It was all about what I needed to do to avoid weight gain. And that day, it meant I needed to run all seven slices of cake off as soon as I could.

Running allowed me to live two different lives--both of which seemed fulfilling at the time. I could make bad nutrition choices, eat way too much food, and still be thin. On paper, I loved it! In reality, binge eating made me feel sick, guilty, and unsatisfied. It was unpredictable and left me out of control.

The disorder also took time away from my family and the things I loved. My long runs took place on Saturday mornings, consisting of anywhere from 15 to 20 miles. One specific morning I remember going to the high school track to run. Afterwards, I texted my wife and asked if she wanted to meet at Ryan's (a favorite!) for breakfast. We made a plan to meet at a certain time, and I knew right then I was going to overeat. So I ran the last 13 miles of that run at a seven minute pace. I wanted to burn as many calories as I could.

We met after my run, and I ate and ate and ate. I ate so much that it ruined the rest of my day. I went home and slept while my family went to a birthday party, watched football, and enjoyed the rest of the afternoon together, but not me. I was lethargic and upset with myself. I didn't feel normal, and I wanted so badly to feel normal. I wanted to be someone who could run, enjoy life, and not overeat to a point where I felt miserable. I wanted to stop, but I didn't know how I could.

I was becoming someone I didn't want to be, and Eddie was right there, encouraging me along. When I wavered, he was right there to remind me how much I wanted to be skinny and how much I had to keep running to be that way.

By this point, I had figured out a formula for my binge eating episodes. It usually took three days to get back to my former weight. During those days I would run more miles and eat less calories. I would restrict my calories to 1600 and run 30-40 miles in three days. This formula usually worked to get me back to my former weight. However, all these workouts had to be done on a treadmill. Running inside allowed me to sweat more and more sweat meant less weight. Sometimes I would be too afraid to weigh myself after those binge sessions, but I knew usually after the third day of my formula I would be back to my former weight.

As I prepared for the Jacksonville marathon, I was steadily losing weight. I worked hard to develop what I thought was the perfect formula to help me run it under three hours. Most days looked the same. Sarah and I had two kids at this point, and, as she was a kindergarten teacher, I worked from home to keep the kids while she was away at school. When they got up, I would fix them breakfast and get ready to run. If it were an easy day, we'd do a quick four to five miles through the neighborhood. If it were a speed or tempo day, we would head to the gym. I rarely took rest days because it was such a mental struggle for me to do so, but when I did, I didn't eat much. On those days, I lowered my caloric intake to between 600 and 800 for the day. But the worse part about off days was the mental battle. I was constantly hungry and thirsty and that made me grumpy and tough on those around me. I was fighting hard not to give in to the temptation to eat or drink more than I had calculated.

At this point I my formula was: eat breakfast, run to eliminate those calories, skip lunch, and then eat dinner with my family. Usually dinner meal was very large, and skipping meals allowed me to bank calories in advance. I looked at dinner as an experience, and this added a lot of pressure to my wife. I put a lot of focus on dinner and wanted the food to be good because I was hungry! My body was craving food, and the hope of dinner consumed my thoughts throughout the day. I looked online at nutrition charts for places I would suggest for dinner. I would research calorie counts of foods so I would be close to knowing how much I was putting in my body I had to know how many calories to expect in order to ease my anxiety. If I didn't know what I was eating or how many calories to anticipate, I was stressed.

My obsession with food became a frequent argument with my wife. I would ask her where she wanted to go for dinner or what she wanted me to cook. I began to take over the cooking responsibilities. Seems like every woman's dream! Not so much. I took it over because I had to know all the ingredients in the food. I didn't want butter because of the fat. I didn't want anything that would cause weight gain. If food wasn't something I felt like I had full control over I would get mad. She couldn't understand why I reacted this way. It was frustrating for her and rightfully so.

Looking back, it was a miracle that I made it to race day. I say that because of my health. I felt healthy because I was running faster than ever before, but I didn't know if my body could take three hours of running. I knew I wasn't properly taking care of my body. No one could convince me that I needed to lift weights to be a stronger runner, eat protein to be healthier, or even drink more water. What mattered most was the number on the scale.

I gave the Jacksonville Bank marathon all I had, and thankfully it was enough. You would have thought reaching my goal was the greatest thing to ever happen. And while I was very excited and proud of my accomplishment, there was still Eddie. I wanted him to go away. I wanted him to leave me alone. And after this race, I really thought he would. I had assured friends and family that I would gain weight and eat more after the marathon. It proved to be much easier said than done. I remember it being less than an hour after I crossed the finish line before Eddie's voice came back and said, "What are you going to do now? You aren't going to run for three days! You better be careful. Here comes the weight gain!"

That night at The Cheesecake Factory I was consumed with fear. I knew I wasn't going to run and so I was worried about what to eat. I was frustrated that I couldn't just celebrate and eat like a person should. I had worked so hard to get to this point, and I thought it would be the end of the frustration and struggle. But it was only the beginning.

Mile

14

I'm going to Disney World

It was Monday after my victory at the Jacksonville Bank Marathon, and my family and I were heading to Disney World for two nights to celebrate.

You might think I would still be riding high on cloud nine, but that wasn't the case. It was a struggle to eat. I kept having thoughts of my running progress--the hard work I'd put in to meet my goal at the race fresh on my mind. And with it, that same thought: if I'm not running, should I even be eating? Not eating sounded crazy, but eating whatever I wanted without running sounded even crazier to me.

I needed a plan.

That shouldn't be a problem. I had operated on a strict plan for the past year of my life. I knew what it took. So I decided to structure my eating schedule just like I did my running schedule. If it worked to get the running results I wanted, why wouldn't it do the same for weight? I decided the first step was to know exactly what went into my body.

If I could predict that, I could predict the results I thought I wanted to see.

When we arrived at the hotel, my wife asked about lunch. I replied quickly that I wasn't hungry but would willingly grab something for her and our daughter, Georgia Grace. She obliged, and I was instantly relieved. Only a few hours into the trip and I had successfully avoided my first meal with unpredictable calories.

After lunch, we headed to the park. Disney World is magical for anyone, but nothing beats taking your child for the first time! It gave me so much joy to see my kids' excitement at all things Mickey Mouse.

Each time we passed a food option, I would stare in and wish I could enjoy it. My mind was torn in two--one half was hungry and screaming at me to eat while the other half was reminding me that I wasn't running and needed to watch myself. Besides, if I ate that food I wouldn't know for sure how many calories I was consuming. I couldn't predict how my body would respond. I wouldn't know the number.

And that wasn't part of the plan.

My daily diet at Disney World consisted of oatmeal: two packets for breakfast, one for lunch, and two for dinner. It may seem a little odd, but it was the only thing available that was pre-packaged. I knew exactly how many calories were going into my body when I ate it so I thought I would be able to predict exactly how my body would respond to it.

I didn't factor in the calories I was burning walking around the parks all day. I wanted more, but I couldn't bring myself to ignore what Eddie was telling me.

And so for three days, it was oatmeal.

Each meal suggestion from Sarah was met with the same response: "You guys go ahead. I'll just eat something here in the hotel." My unwillingness to eat was making Sarah upset. She was starting to see that maybe I did, in fact, have a problem. She wanted to enjoy more of the meals while we were there, but I didn't. I couldn't. I couldn't eat knowing that I had to weigh in when I got home. I couldn't destroy all the hard work that I had put in to get to this point. What I didn't understand at that time was that not eating was destroying my body. I was slowly going into a downward spiral that would cost me years of hard work.

The true test for me would come on Wednesday when we returned home. I would weigh again--my first time since completing the race. Three days without running should only gain me a few pounds, right? That would be okay. It wouldn't take long to lose it once I was back home. The thought of even gaining a little weight was frightening. The scale consumed my mind at all times.

Looking back I realize my lack of energy and frustration during that trip was my body's way of telling me that what I was doing wasn't healthy. It was sending me all the warning signals I needed, but I was brushing them off. Eddie had convinced me that what I thought was right wasn't the truth. There was no middle ground with him. If I wasn't running, I couldn't eat. That's what he told me, and that's what I believed.

Mile

15

Weigh in

As we arrived home, I prepared myself to face the inevitable weigh in. After previous marathons, I would see a weight gain of about one pound per day post race. Taking this into consideration I prepared myself for at least a three-pound gain from three days off running. Weighing in was all I thought about on the drive home. I was mentally trying to prepare myself for what I would see.

My lowest weight preparing for the Jacksonville marathon was 126 pounds. Those last few weeks leading up to the race I saw consistent and rapid weight loss of about one pound per week. That's not drastic for marathon preparation, but at my weight, it was significant. I was running faster than I ever had before, and I thought the explanation was simple: the smaller my body, the faster the run.

I projected my weight on race day to be around 128 pounds.

But what would the number be now?

I undressed and stepped on the scale in our bathroom when I got home. Undressing was a standard for me when weighing in. I didn't want anything to influence the scale in one direction or the other. I wanted to make sure I eliminated anything that would sway the scale. I watched the numbers circle with anxiety before landing on my weight.

124.4.

What? How could that be? I didn't run for three days and had somehow lost weight! I stepped on to the scale and then back off again. There it was again: 124.4.

And just like that, all of my anxiety seemed to leave. I had survived. Three days without running, and I didn't blow up into an unfit hot air balloon. I had won. Strangely the number on the scale brought me more excitement than three days at Disney World. It was pitiful. How could I have fallen so far and become so enslaved to the scale?

There was nothing about my food choices that were even close to healthy. I had restricted my diet at the sacrifice of my energy level and family. To say it was consuming is an understatement. Eddie and the scale controlled my life.

In that moment, my thinking shifted. I don't think I even realized it at the time, but right then, I decided that the number on the scale determined my perception of myself.

It didn't matter what I saw in the mirror, how I felt, what others said. It didn't even matter how my runs went. If the number on the scale increased, I had done something wrong. I had failed. But if that number went down, I was doing something right. I was on track.

I knew what I needed to do to stay on track.

The reality is that numbers formed my perception of myself. That's an incredibly unhealthy way to perceive myself. There is no reason why a number on the scale should form my confidence, identity, or worth. But at that time, it was. No longer was my performance defined by how well I ran during a workout or race. My performance, what I ate, and when I ate were all determined by the number on the scale. If the number was higher, it meant I had eaten too much or didn't exercise enough. To me, a high number on the scale showed me to be weak, but a low number meant I was in control. It meant I was strong. The scale controlled my emotions, my self-perception, and my actions.

I shared some of my faith earlier in this book because it was one of the pillars that helped me during my recovery. I learned to rest in the fact that my identity is truly found in my Savior, Jesus Christ. There is nothing that I can do--no race I can run and no number I can achieve--that will ever make God love me more than He does now. He loves me no matter what and that's the foundation of my identity.

Mile

16

A new routine

My passion for running slowly started to dwindle along with my energy level. It just wasn't fun anymore. I was becoming apathetic towards so many things in my life. It was a symptom of the disorder taking over my life. It felt like things just didn't matter anymore.

At first I wrote this newfound apathy off as normal--a simple case of the post-marathon blues. Wasn't it normal to see my excitement for the sport diminish a little with no race to train for on the horizon? I figured the excitement would return when I found a new race or set a new goal.

But the truth was, I knew this was more than a simple case of the blues. It wasn't normal. I didn't like running anymore because it had become simply a means to an end. I didn't want to run anymore, and I certainly didn't have the energy for it. I just wanted to be skinny. If you were to have asked me which mattered more to me at the time--being skinny or having enough energy to run--I would have said without a doubt that it was being skinny. I needed to stay healthy and to stay healthy I had to stay skinny.

In my mind, I equated being healthy to being skinny, but in reality, there was nothing healthy about how skinny I was. Oh how easily the devil can deceive us!

Even though I didn't feel like it, I ran. I continued to run as if I were training and monitored my calorie intake like never before. I began a new routine designed to keep me skinny.

Each day I got up and ate two packets of oatmeal before starting work for the day. Oatmeal had quickly become a staple in my diet as it allowed me to know exactly what was going into my body. It was predictable and easy. It was routine. I didn't want to eat anything else, and if I did, it needed to be pre-packaged.

After the kids woke up, I would fix breakfast, and, out of habit, usually finished off a few bites of whatever they left behind. It was after this that the guilt usually began to set in. Why did I let myself eat their breakfast? Why couldn't I just stop with the oatmeal?

Always after the guilt came the run. I got the kids ready and rushed to the gym. We typically arrived daily around 10:30 each morning and with the kid's care not closing until 1:00, I could get in a solid two-hour workout.

The goal during those workouts was simple: to burn off my morning's calories and then some.

I hoped to see 1,000 calories off by the end of my morning workouts. This would get rid of my breakfast calories as well as bank some additional calories for the rest of the day. How well I did on those morning workouts determined what I would allow myself to eat for the rest of the day. If I didn't run as well I didn't eat as much. That was the formula.

But the formula was laced with guilt and fear. I didn't want to run that far anymore. I wanted to enjoy more time with my kids, but unfortunately my addiction was continuously taking away from my family and my health. The exhaustion after these runs was horrible. I wanted to play with my kids instead of running so long. I wanted to concentrate on work but I couldn't. All I thought about was the next time I would weigh

Around 2:00pm everyday our babysitter would arrive, and I'd head into work for a couple of hours. I had just organized an after school running program call Run Hard. The program coached kids on the sport of running and also taught character values that would help them understand their potential. The program was very rewarding because it allowed me to see running influence young kids the same way it had influenced me. I wish at the time I had been a better role model for how to keep your body healthy. But I was too sick to see what I was doing to myself. Since then I've learned valuable lessons that have benefited the program and allowed me to better lead the kids. I've continued to say that I wish there was Run Hard for me when I was in elementary school.

But then, the routine continued. Day in and day out, I would eat only when I could run. The scale drove me.

I monitored my weight by stepping onto the scale multiple times a day. I would get up in the morning and weigh in. I would eat breakfast, take a shower, and weigh in. I would weigh after the gym, after a meal, after work. I was a slave to the numbers.

And that's really how I felt: like I was in prison. I had no identity. I was controlled by something else--owned by the numbers. They dictated everything about my life. I see now that it was really a deception of the devil holding me hostage. And it happened without me even knowing.

I didn't wake up one day and decide I was going to stop eating. I didn't just cut my diet or increase my workouts overnight. It was a slow and gradual process. I slowly removed God from the throne of my life and replaced Him with something else--with the lies of the devil in the shape of the numbers on the scale. Eddie's voice was constantly telling me that what I was doing was right--a factor that only contributed to my downfall.

The disease had changed everything about me. Even my family felt the change. Preparation for meals brought so much tension between my wife and me. I needed to know everything we would be eating that week before it happened. I couldn't be taken by surprise. If we were going out to eat, I needed to know days in advance to prepare my body for the additional calorie intake. Preparation for going out to eat meant I would fast and restrict myself even more so that I could eat a normal meal in public. Nothing involving food could happen on a whim for me anymore. Date nights were miserable. I would cause arguments because of the inability to make food choices.

And that's because food was no longer a source of pleasure for me. I didn't see it as fuel for my body. Food was a reward for a hard workout. Food was something I had to earn. And by earn, I mean run. If I ate, I had to have a run before and a run after. It almost became a challenge for me. I would try to research and guess how many calories my food had in it, and then workout as hard as I could to see if I could zero out those calories.

If it sounds miserable, that's because it was. I truly was sick, but I didn't fully realize it yet.

Mile

17

Downward spiral

By late January of 2013, I was consumed with my new routine, and my body showed it.

I was at my lowest weight yet: 118.6.

I remember the day I saw this number on the scale. It was after an extremely hard morning workout designed to bank some calories for my daughter's birthday dinner that night at a pizza buffet. As the number flashed on the scale, a thought crept in with it: *That doesn't seem healthy.*

I quickly shook my head in hopes to shake the thought from my mind, and it worked. I pushed it out and replaced it with celebration. This low number meant I had earned my dinner. I could eat. I remember skipping lunch even though I was very hungry because I couldn't bring myself to eat if it meant sacrificing any of the calories I had banked for dinner. This disordered thinking would allow me the feeling of freedom when it came to dinner. I knew I wouldn't be able to have control over my eating at dinner so I needed to make sure I had enough calories "saved" before I ate. That meant avoiding eating or drinking anything for the rest of the day. During mealtimes after a short fast I would be so hungry. I would eat fast and overeat. Then I would feel the guilt and start the running routine over again. Eat, run, eat. I hated it. I wanted to eat normal portions and not be slave to the thinking that I had to run after each meal.

Limiting water was a new restriction for me. As a runner, you're taught how important hydration is for your body, but somewhere along the way I decided that this too was not necessary. Even water added weight, and weight was bad. If the scale told me I couldn't eat, why couldn't it tell me that I couldn't drink either?

Regulating my water intake took the harm to my body to a new level, and I saw it in full effect during a business trip to St. Louis. I was in St. Louis attending a conference for my job--a conference that included lavish meals provided by the hosts. In order to allow myself to partake in any of these meals, I would get up early and run 12 miles on the indoor treadmill. I dressed for warmth for those runs, hoping to sweat off even more weight during the workout. Because I had no scale with me during the trip, I felt the pressure to workout even harder. It was the only way I knew to do it.

The last day of the conference I ran on the treadmill for a late afternoon workout. I had a buffet lunch with two trips to the dessert bar prior to that, and the guilt from that meal motivated me to run. I completed my 12 miles to burn off my lunch calories and returned to the locker room. There, I noticed something new: there was blood in my urine.

That had never happened before. I was obviously alarmed, but as I was going home the next day, I decided to put off the panic. If it continued to happen, I would handle it back home.

By the time I did get home, the blood was no longer there. I shook it off as something I ate and decided to move on. As I updated Sarah on my trip, I opted to leave out that detail. Why worry her over what was probably nothing?

The next day I tried to settle back into my routine. I would get up, eat breakfast, and go to the gym. However, breakfast didn't go as planned. I hadn't run the previous day so I didn't eat much and woke up very hungry as a result. I ate my regular breakfast, but quickly ate noticed that I still had most of the St. Louis butter cake I brought home with me! It was a treat I brought home for my wife, but that morning, with most of the cake remaining, I ate the entire thing. I wanted to stop, but I just kept telling myself it would only be one more small slice. I couldn't stop. There was nothing I could do. I didn't have the willpower to stop the binge eating.

After the cake was finished, I was left with a huge amount of guilt. I couldn't believe that I had eaten the entire cake! I knew then that I had to make the next workout tough-- almost a punishment on myself for the mistake I made with breakfast. I wanted to have control over my eating, but I couldn't. I was mad at myself and needed to do whatever I could at the gym to work off the extra calories consumed.

As I arrived at the gym, I was eager to complete my workout. While I was away on business I couldn't workout as hard as I normally did, and as I ran that first day home, I felt great. My entire run continued to quicken as I closed in on an hour tempo run. With two miles of warm-up followed by an hour tempo run, I was getting close to 11.5 miles for the day.

During that entire run the thoughts of my binge eating that morning played over in my mind. I could hear Eddie telling me to push harder because of what I'd done. I was miserable over what I'd done, but felt better with every mile run. As I ran, I felt my level of anxiety of the binge eating slowly begin to go down.

Back in the locker room after my run, I stopped in to use the bathroom before picking up the kids. As I went to flush, I noticed something horrifying: a deep garnet pool of blood. My urine was nothing but blood.

At this point, I was truly scared. I had no idea what was happening, but knew I needed to see a doctor. And fast!

The rest of that week consisted of numerous visits to the doctor, tests, scans, and ultrasounds to find the source of my problem. Each one returned normal. There seemed to be nothing major in my body causing the problem. An appointment with a urologist finally confirmed that to be true. It wasn't something *in* my body causing the issue; it was something my body was missing.

Water.

I was so dehydrated that the walls of my bladder were rubbing together as I ran, causing me to bleed. The doctor's orders were clear: stop running and start drinking.

Stop running?!? That felt like a death sentence to me. If I did that, I was sure to gain weight. But I recognized what the doctor said had to be true. If I didn't want that to keep happening, I had to make some changes.

Unfortunately I decided to make changes to the wrong things. If I couldn't run, I had to change the way I was eating. I started cutting out small things in my diet (like milk from my cereal) to avoid any unnecessary calories. I read nutrition labels like they were the Bible. I would calculate, measure, and weigh everything that went into my body. I had to know the exact number of calories I was consuming since I couldn't burn any off with running. This addition to my lifestyle only escalated the misery. I had to calculate everything.

But as long as the number on the scale was going down, I felt like I was doing something right.

By April I was running again. Not because I wanted to and not because I missed it, but because I felt obligated to do it. It was simply a means to an end.

It was only a short time until I saw 118.6 again. However, this time I wasn't as impressed. I'd seen that number before and Eddie had convinced me that maintaining my weight wasn't acceptable. I had to lose weight at all costs in order to avoid failure.

But at 118.6, that thought scared me to action.

I decided I needed to tell someone the truth, and my chosen someone was Toby. Toby was a long time friend and mentor so I figured he would be the right person. It was hard to muster the courage to tell him what I had secretly known for a while: I had a problem.

I didn't tell Sarah at first because I didn't want to burden her with what I was going through. My actions were already tough enough for her to deal with that I didn't want to add anything else to her plate. Besides, I didn't yet have a plan. When I told Sarah, I wanted to have a plan to reassure her that I was going to get better. As a husband, I didn't want to make my wife question how well I would be able to provide for her.

Of course she was already questioning if I was going to be okay. She didn't vocalize this to me often because it usually lead to an argument. I was afraid that if I were to open up to her without a plan of action, she would have questions that I didn't know how to answer. I wanted her to feel safe and secure in the face of my disease--something I didn't think could happen without a plan.

So Toby was the first person I opened up to about my illness. I set up a meeting seemingly to discuss work. After the business was out of the way, I blurted out to Toby, "I think I'm killing myself."

And just like that, it was out there.

I was completely transparent with Toby, sharing with him everything that had been going on in my life and in my head over the last few months. Being transparent with someone is very important and a great first step for me. I didn't know where to turn, what to do, but I knew I had to tell someone.

He responded by encouraging me to get help. He even researched a few places to go for counseling. I had never been to a counselor before and, come to think of it, had never really asked for help with any tough situation I'd encountered.

I was nervous, but it felt like a step in the right direction.

Mile

18

Getting help

The initial phone call to the counselor was scary. What if the person on the other end of the line recognized my voice? What if I saw someone I knew in the waiting room? I'm a guy; what's a guy doing calling an eating disorder clinic? I mean, I wasn't even sure I had an eating disorder. What would they think if they saw me there? No one else knew what was going on in my life except for my wife and Toby (at least that's what I told myself).

As I've gotten distance from this time in my life and shared some of my story with others, I'm often surprised by just how much many people in my life already knew. Even though I believed I was hiding it, they could all tell just by looking at me. They all knew something was wrong, maybe even before I did! But it was hard for them to voice any of their concerns to me. It's hard to confront friends and relatives when you see something they're doing that's destroying them. A confrontation can jeopardize the relationship and that's not something most people feel comfortable risking. They all wanted to help, but they didn't know how.

The day of my appointment arrived, and as Sarah and I drove to the office, my anxiety steadily increased. When I made the appointment I told Sarah about my conversation with Toby. I told her I felt like I had a problem, and she agreed. She was glad I was looking for help, and she wanted to be there to support me. My initial revelation about my disease brought her to tears. I didn't realize how much pain I had caused her during those past few years and months. Seeing her emotional response game me a little more incentive to take the first step to getting better. But as the time drew near for me to go to counseling, I tried to find ways to get out of it. I didn't want to go. If I could have turned around and never had to answer to my wife or Toby about it, I would have.

But I was stuck.

The entire first appointment felt uncomfortable. I was riddled with guilt and embarrassment but deep down knew I needed to be there. The counselor began by saying, "So Jesse, tell me what's going on."

That seemed simple.

And so I started talking. I told her about running and how much I used to love it. I told her about the scale and how it ruled my life. I was weighing myself nearly ten times a day at that point. I told her about my routine and the way I watched my eating. As I finished talking, she asked me my current weight.

It was around 122 at that point.

When I said it aloud, her eyebrows immediately raised. Then she shifted her focus to Sarah.

She asked my wife to describe me a little. She wanted to know about our trip to Disney, how Sarah felt not being able to go out to eat, and how my running impacted her life.

And just like that, the floodgates opened for Sarah.

She wept as she transparently shared her feelings with the counselor. She told her how emotionless I'd become--how completely detached she felt I was from the family. She saw no emotion in me, no desire to be with her, and no emotional investment in our family. And the worst part? She was right. Deep down, none of that mattered to me as much as the scale.

The counselor began to describe me to Sarah as if she knew me. She told Sarah things I would do, things I would think, things I would say--all without me even telling her. It was as if she'd jumped inside my mind and given the most accurate description of all that was going on in there at the time.

Turns out, she wasn't describing Jesse Harmon.

She was describing a person suffering from Anorexia Nervosa. She was describing Eddie.

And that's who I had become.

She turned to me then and described my condition to me directly. She told me that she specialized in the disease, having helped many others find recovery, and she wanted to help me do the same. She described in detail how the disease worked, how every person suffering from it has a limit. Once that person passes their limit, it's like a point of no return. The brain deceives the body into believing that it's gaining weight and that nothing can be done to stop it. I was in this category of deception, but she believed I could still be cured.

Cured.

I found myself hung up on that word. What did she mean by that?

"Jesse," she said in response, "you're dying. And I'm trying to save your life."

She went on to explain that she believed the best course of action was admittance into a 30-day program at an inpatient facility that specialized in treating patients with anorexia. There would be hurdles, with few facilities accepting male patients and even fewer insurance companies agreeing to cover the stay, but she thought it was absolutely necessary.

I was stunned. None of this was what I expected. I had planned to come to this counseling session just to talk, and all of the sudden she says I'm sick. And dying. And the only way to fix it is to leave my family for at least 30 days?

I resisted. It was the truth, but I was still fighting it.

I left in disbelief. My world flipped in two hours. I left overwhelmed. Quickly Eddie started talking, reassuring me that I wasn't anorexic and I wasn't dying. I was just a runner who had gotten off his plan and needed to start running again to get things back to they way they were.

And instead of the counselor, I chose to listen to Eddie.

Mile

19

The plan

Lucky for me, Sarah has always been a rule follower. When the counselor said come up with a plan, Sarah was going to make sure we did just that. We decided on a plan that we were both comfortable with. We would go to counseling together twice a week and talk about some possible next steps. Then we would work together to make sure I followed the counselor's recommendations. This would substitute for me going to a facility. I figured I could do it this way if I applied all of my willpower. If this worked, I wouldn't need an inpatient facility.

My next meeting with the counselor included a nutritionist. My greatest fear at that meeting was the weigh in. I knew the nutritionist would record my weight, and as I hadn't been running as much since starting counseling, I knew I would see a gain in my weight. In a way, it was as if my greatest fear was coming true: I was gaining weight and powerless to stop it.

I waited in the lobby amongst three other women. This was the first time I truly began to feel awkward in my situation. I was the only man in what felt like a sea of women. I was fighting what was typically known to be a woman's disease. Of course I know now that anorexia can hit anyone--man or woman. But at the time, my impression of the disease was based on the elementary knowledge I had of it. At the time, it was hard to find information or testimony about men struggling the way I was.

Sitting in the waiting room I listened as the women talked with one another about their meal plans. They shared how much food they ate, the charts they were given by the nutritionist to record their meals, and how much hesitation they had to eat anything at all. Listening to them was like listening to the voices inside my head. It was exactly how I had been living. As I heard them talk, I knew that I didn't want to be that person anymore. Their rational sounded wrong; I knew what they were saying was not true. It was a clear picture of who I had become.

Once the nutritionist called me back to her office, she immediately started in with a line of questioning. How much did I eat? What did I eat? What did I drink? She listened and recorded each of my answers meticulously.

And then came the weigh in. I had planned ahead for this by trying to wear clothes that were as light as possible to avoid any extra weight on the scale. This was just another example of how much the scale and numbers controlled me. I thought about it for days. I tried to plan my reaction to any weight gain. The scale brought fear and anxiety, and as I stepped up to the scale, I removed my shoes and my shirt. I didn't care what it took; I just wanted that number to be as low as possible.

And there it was: 127.

At first, I was just relieved to finally know the number. I hadn't weighed myself in the days since counseling so even though I was discouraged to see weight gain, I was excited to finally know my weight. Part of our plan was that I couldn't weigh myself outside the counselor's office. Not at the gym, not at the house, not at all. We still had a scale at the house, but I wanted to show both Sarah and myself that I had the self-discipline not to use it. But now that I knew the number, I knew exactly what I had to do next: lower it.

The nutritionist ended our appointment by letting me know that she would be emailing me a meal plan. She wanted me to follow that menu exactly. And deep down, I wanted to at least try to do as she asked. A part of me was screaming for help, and I was trying as hard as I could to listen to that voice instead of Eddie's.

I attempted to follow the meal plan, but it ended up being very difficult for me. Before the meal plan, I was binge eating calories and burning them off in a pattern. The meal plan meant no more binging. Instead, it laid out what exactly what I needed to eat and how much. For example, breakfast would consist of two carbs, one protein, and a starch of some sort. Each part of the plan included a number representing how many grams of each I was supposed to eat. The nutritionist obviously meant for the best when outlining my meal plan, but the numbers listed there again attempted to control my life. The meal plan opened a new way to live by the numbers.

For the first couple of weeks, I followed the plan closely. I wanted to get better, and the meal plan seemed like the first step to getting there. However, I quickly realized that the food on the meal plan wasn't enough for me. I continued to weigh in secretly while on the meal plan, and noticed I was losing weight. I should have let my nutritionist know this so she could modify my plan, but I liked the fact that I was losing weight without a run. For me, it was a win!

Only a few weeks into counseling, I started running again. I convinced myself that since I was trying to get healthy, running for my health couldn't be bad. I thought I could manage. But with running, I was burning every calorie I consumed on the meal plan. I rationalized my habits as moderation. I was only eating a little and running a little. That couldn't be bad, right?

Running brought the scale back to my life in full force. I was weighing myself again regularly and monitoring my progress by the number. The scale became my fix. I had loads of anxiety from not weighing, but once I weighed in and knew the number, everything was okay.

The meal plan allowed me to monitor my weight closer than ever (not the result the nutritionist was looking for). The more I followed the plan in combination with running, the lower my weight would drop.

And just like that, the new plan was forgotten.

Mile

20

Intervention

After only four visits, I made the decision to stop going to counseling. I felt like it wasn't helping me, and it seemed like a lot of money to spend on something that wasn't working. It wasn't working because of my decisions. I wasn't listening to their advice. I wasn't doing what they asked me to do to get better. Sarah asked why I stopped going, and I told her the counselor was saying the same stuff over and over. I assured her that I knew what to do and that getting better was up to me.

The truth is counseling could've helped me, but I wasn't committed to it. I wasn't committed to anything that made me feel better. I believed I had everything under control-- that I could change whenever I wanted to change. I was still running, still weighing in, and still eating less and less. And I felt fine.

In June of 2013 I got a call from Toby asking me to meet with him and Todd, the pastor of our church, for a chat. I agreed to sit down with them both that week. Toby didn't have to say what the chat would be about; I already knew.

Other people in my life were already doing the same thing. They would call me up, ask to meet, and then share their concerns about my weight. I would assure them everything was fine, that I'd been seeing a counselor and had even started to gain weight. None of this was true of course, but it got me out of the conversation.

As soon as I sat down with Todd and Toby, that same conversation began to play out. They asked me questions, they shared their concerns, and I answered by trying to explain the situation. As they were closer to me than most, I did share a little more with them than I had with others.

When I finished my explanation, Todd replied simply, "You sound like an addict."

That response caught me completely off guard. It was the first time anyone had ever called me that, but something about it resonated with me. It almost sounded right.

He continued, "Addicts don't get healthy without help. We're here to tell you tonight that you have to get help. You have to go to treatment. There are no other choices."

I was completely speechless. I felt numb. This was the first time anyone had ever laid down such an ultimatum to me. I found myself agreeing to talk to my wife about it and quickly getting out of the room.

124

I barely made it a mile away from the church before having to pull over. I felt like a zombie. I was stunned at what had just happened. Did I just agree to go to a facility? Was I actually going to have to do it? How did it get this far? What was I going to say to my family?

By the time I made it home, Sarah was waiting eagerly to find out how the meeting had gone. I didn't sugar coat it. I didn't have the energy. I just plopped down into our recliner and blurted out, "They're making me leave."

And then I lost it.

I felt like the weight of the world was sitting on my shoulders, crushing me at that point. The weight of people knowing the truth of my condition, the weight of wondering who was going to take care of everything while I was away. The weight of missing my family for at least a month, all that weight was too heavy to hold, and my emotions gave way. I couldn't hold them in any more.

Georgia Grace and Graham were playing nearby, and, seeing me upset, promptly crawled into my lap. Isn't it funny how children do that? They don't need to know why; they just know you need comfort. Eventually Sarah joined us, and together our little family sat there and held one another. I'll be honest, it was a little tough to breathe with three people sitting on my lap! But it was the perfect reminder of all I had to live for and work for in recovery.

After a few minutes, we broke apart and reality set back in. Sarah and I began the process of researching a facility. We spent the next few hours calling those that would accept male patients (that list isn't long) before settling on a place in the middle of Florida. We talked to the admissions counselor, gathering all the details about the requirements for the program. And finally, the bottom line: this program would cost $60,000. In that moment, as much as we wanted to, Sarah and I knew we couldn't pay for it.

But I also knew that I couldn't return to Todd and Toby without a plan that resembled something like it. So I developed a plan.

At the time, we had limited income and operated on a pretty strict food budget. This plan threw that out the window. The goal was to have any food that I was willing to eat. In the beginning, if I wanted to go out to eat every night at my favorite restaurant, that's what we'd do. We knew it was going to cost more money than we had allotted for the month, but the sacrifice in funds we hoped would lead to healing.

The plan also included counseling. I would have to go to counseling to make sure I was on the right path. I had to check in twice a week to make sure I was gaining weight, eating, and discussing my struggles with a counselor.

Todd and Toby demanded that I stop running, and I agreed to it. No running. No matter how much I tried to rationalize the reason for my running, I couldn't. There was no good reason for me to run (unless it was to save a life).

In the back of my mind I knew that wouldn't be a problem. I had learned how to count calories, to portion my meals, and control my eating. If I couldn't lose weight running, I would do it another way. The truth is Todd was right: I was an addict. I was addicted to the numbers. I was addicted to losing weight. And if they took away one way for me to do it, I would find something else.

Even though the plan I'd laid out for them was strong, my addiction was stronger. And I walked forward into the summer of 2013 as a suffering and struggling addict.

Mile

21

Summer of 2013

By the time summer approached, I had completely stopped running. It was more of a chore to me than anything else at that point--a punishment to my body for consuming too many calories. Besides, I had promised Todd and Toby I would give it up, and I wanted to do my best to keep that promise.

However, I was still hearing Eddie's voice nonstop. I wasn't supposed to weigh anymore, but he encouraged me to find new ways to measure my weight. I would wear the same belt and note how my pants fit each day. I would pay close attention to certain areas of my body and try to notice any differences (something I had never done before). I was using the way my body looked to try and gauge my weight.

Eddie also made sure I was aware of what I was eating, constantly reminding me of what I shouldn't be putting into my body. I was still obsessively controlling everything that went into my body. I researched calorie counts, measured all my food, and carefully portioned everything that went into my body. If we were going out to eat, I would spend hours researching the available calorie counts online for the restaurant. I was slowly removing entire food groups from my diet to try and lower my calorie intake. First it was milk. Then it was salad dressings. Then it was carbs. Whatever it took, I was going to make sure I was in control of my calories.

Things quickly spiraled downward. Soon my breakfast consisted of one apple sliced with salt and pepper and a diet soda. Carbonated diet drinks had become a staple in my diet. They made me feel full without the calories. At times I would drink up to seven cans a day just to trick my body into believing it was full. The feeling was horrible. I would be dizzy from the carbonated drinks. I wouldn't have any energy to play with my kids. I was miserable and struggling to change. No matter how lethargic I felt, it didn't compare to the fear of gaining weight.

And of course, I started to weigh myself regularly again. I was still a slave to the scale.
It's like I became a zombie. I had no energy and no emotions. To say I was making life miserable for my family would be an understatement. They were living with the shell of the person I used to be. I was not the person that Sarah married. I no longer had any drive to do anything. Nothing else seemed to matter; all I wanted to do was to continue to lose weight.

That summer we made a trip to visit Sarah's family in Kentucky. I was riddled with anxiety about leaving the

129

house and being so far away from the scale. But if my regimented eating program had taught me anything it was how to control the number. I knew exactly what I needed to eat (or not eat as the case may be) in order to avoid weight gain--even if I didn't have the scale to confirm it. I became even more destructive when I was away from the scale, restricting myself more because of the fear of gaining weight.

We celebrated my birthday while on that family trip to Kentucky. But for me, instead of a celebration, it was more of a cause to worry. I knew Sarah would want to take me out, and her family would make a cake. I had to do something to prepare.

So on my birthday, I decided I would treat myself to a run. I thought it would be both a great way to bank some calories before the big dinner tonight as well as see if I still had it in me to push through a run.

I didn't know what the run would look like, but I expected it to be rough. I decided start slow: run one minute, walk one minute, repeat as long as I could. The thought of running a mile without stopping felt like climbing a mountain. I had not run since early June, and my muscle mass had rapidly declined alongside my weight. I knew a run would hurt.

And it did. As I planned, I ran one minute then stopped for one minute. I did six reps like this before having to stop completely. I could barely finish six minutes without needing to rest! I couldn't believe how far I had fallen. Just eight months prior I ran a marathon averaging 6:48 per mile and now I could hardly jog for six minutes.

I was destroyed in every way. Physically, mentally, emotionally--the disease and deception had taken it all. I realized in those six minutes that what I was doing was damaging my body in every way. But even still, the hold on my mind was strong and a part of me didn't even care. I cared more about the scale than the reality I was facing.

I told myself I wanted to get better, but I couldn't make myself eat.

I eventually made it back to the house, unsatisfied with my run and the lack of calories burned. That evening's birthday meal was sure to be a challenge.

Really, every meal was a challenge at that point. I would see how small of a meal I could eat, and if I ate smaller, I won. Eating small meant fewer calories and fewer calories meant beating the scale. Restriction allowed me to feel a sense of control, and control is what I liked.

I had completely abandoned my plan for recovery at that point. Sure, I wasn't running, but as I'd just discovered, I couldn't run if I wanted to at that point. I wasn't going to counseling anymore. I wasn't consuming the recommended calories. I wasn't doing any of it.

Mile

22

Rock bottom

Eventually I had to tell the rest of my family what I was going through. I knew my parents and brother suspected something was wrong, but they didn't have a clue how severe it really was. I sat down with them and opened up completely, telling them about the diagnosis of anorexia and what the doctor said it was doing to my body. I gave it to them straight: my life was in danger. Telling my family was a way for me to admit to myself that I had a problem. That's why it took so long for me to tell them. I had to be honest with myself and with my family.

Understandably my mom took the situation very hard. She would cry when we talked about it, and was consumed with worry. At one point, she sat me down and shared in detail about a dream she'd had about my kids visiting me in the hospital. I was lying there asleep, and my daughter was shaking me, screaming, "Daddy, wake up!" But in the dream, I never woke up.

You would think conversations like this would cause me to want to change, but it didn't. It was just a dream, and in reality, I felt like I had everything under control. I thought eventually I would get better, but for now, it felt like no one understood what I was going through.

The truth was that I was having similar dreams. I dreamed about dying. I dreamed about my own funeral. I dreamed about my kids' lives without me in them. I wrote each one off as just another dream--something fictional that wouldn't really happen. Looking back I believe God was trying to communicate the truth of my situation to me. These dreams were going to come true if I continued down this path.

I had never been so confused. I knew logically what I was doing to my body, but I couldn't stop. At night I would stand in front of the mirror and stare at the bones sticking out from my skin. I would go to bed with my stomach screaming at me to feed it, so hungry at times I'd wonder if I would even be able to get out of bed the next morning. I was worried about my life constantly. My counselor had told me that in severe cases of anorexia, the heart eventually just stops. The body has nothing left to fuel it, and so it just stops working.

But even that wasn't enough for me to stop. It was a risk I was willing to take.

As a child I used to wonder at times what the devil looked like. Did he have big horns? Was he dressed in all black?

Standing in front of my bathroom mirror, eyes sunken in and bones protruding everywhere, I saw him looking back at me. And it wasn't pretty. My heart was hollow and my spirit was gone. I didn't know what to do. I didn't know how to fix what I had done. How did I get this far?

I truly believe the devil had taken me down a path of deception so dark that I was consumed by it. This addiction had taken me to places I never thought possible, and at the bottom of each of them was the devil. His deception was at the very root of my disease.

I stepped on the scale once more.

112.8.

That was the lowest I had ever seen the number go, and I was terrified. Not just by the number itself. No, I was more afraid of the thought that crossed my mind as soon as I saw it.

That isn't low enough.

And in response to that thought, I said aloud, alone in the bathroom, "I'm dying."

I said it because it was true. I wanted to get better, but I couldn't. I couldn't seem to convince myself that the scale wasn't important. I couldn't seem to make myself eat enough to gain weight. And if I couldn't do those things, I couldn't survive.

Mile

23

The process

The reality that my life was on the line began to motivate me to try and get better for a while. I really believed that I could do it on my own. I really did want to get better, and I thought that was enough.

To fully be released from my addiction, I needed a full surrender. I had to release it all: the running, the eating, and the scale. Until I was ready to do that, I wasn't going to be healed no matter how much weight I allowed myself to gain.

It was now October 2013. Fall had arrived and brought with it a new anxiety. The crispness in the air meant no more sweating. And without running, sweat was the only thing I had to make me feel as though I was burning off calories. I couldn't sweat. I couldn't go outside. It was cold, and I was very intolerant of cold weather. The continuous thought of gaining weight was a burden. There were countless times I would ask myself why I was thinking about my weight. Why couldn't I be normal? I wanted to live life and not think about weight, food, and running all the time.

So slowly, I allowed myself to gain weight. Adding pounds came with complete anxiety. I hated the feeling. Every one-pound gained to me felt like ten. As I gained weight I wondered what others thought. I wondered how big I looked to them. I wondered if people would question my identity as a runner. Being unhealthy and skinny allowed me to play that part. Even though I was in horrible health, I still looked like a runner (at least in my mind).

Though I was beginning to take small steps to look and feel healthier, Eddie was still there. He incessantly whispered what I was doing wrong, how gaining weight would lead me to become the kid I used to be. He reminded me that weight gain meant seclusion and little self-worth. I was so afraid.

Recovery is tough. It takes time and patience, and there is no timetable for each person's personal recovery. Some recover faster than others. Some believe full-recovery isn't a possibility--that it's a lifelong process. I didn't know if recovery was a possibility but I wanted to try.

Giving up the scale was a hard step for me in recovery. In fact it remains the most difficult part of the process today. I was plagued by questions of what would happen to me after the scale. How would I know how much I weighed? If I didn't know how much I weighed, how could I know if I was doing something right? People in my life had long been urging me to give up the scale, and I wanted to do it. I wanted to look at the scale and not care what the number read. I wanted to be able to not look at all. It was going to be a struggle.

Both running and the scale had become negative parts of my life thanks to my disease. In order to hopefully have them be positive again, I had to give them up. I had to stop running in order to one day run again. I had to get rid of the scale in order to eventually one day be to weigh in without care. I had to surrender and do it fully.

In an effort to take a step in the right direction, I asked Sarah to hide the scales. I didn't want to weigh anymore, and I couldn't if I didn't know where they were. She happily agreed.

A couple of days went by without incident before the anxiety hit. The thought of my weight consumed me, and I broke. Like an addict looking for drugs, I ripped the house apart to find the scale. I didn't see Sarah throw it away so I knew it had to be somewhere. The whole time I was looking for it, I knew how wrong it was, but I didn't care. I couldn't stop. I *needed* it. And when I finally found it in the bathroom closet, it was a huge relief.

I took the scale out of the closet and noticed it was out of batteries. She had thrown the batteries away. I was mad. Why did she throw the batteries away? Was it not enough to just hide the scales?

I wouldn't be deterred. I went to the store to buy new batteries. I came back home, quickly weighed myself, returned the scale to its hiding place, and never said a word to anyone.

I knew the whole time that I was not getting better. My rational mind knew I wanted to get better and that I needed help to do it. My actions were full of desperation and deception. This whole incident with the scale proved just how ruled by the disease I still was. I was a prisoner in my own body and mind.

And so this continued for nearly a month. I would wait until I was alone, weigh myself, and return the scale just as I had found it. I thought I was getting away with it--that it was my secret.

Sarah eventually found out what I was doing and confronted me about the scale. She told me how betrayed she felt by this deception. This lie had completely broken her trust, and she was afraid she would never be able to trust me again. If I would lie to her about this, what else would I lie about? She wanted me to get better, but the reality of my secret weigh in communicated to her that I didn't want to get better. My addiction had already broken me down, but now it was breaking down my wife.

I had been telling her that I was getting better, that I was making improvements every day. My actions now showed her otherwise. My sin was taking me farther than I'd ever intended to go, destroying people I never wanted to hurt.

And I was afraid it was about to cost me my marriage.

That conversation with my wife changed everything for me. It woke something up inside of me: the fight. I wanted to fight for my family. I wanted to fight for my marriage. I wanted to fight for my life.

My pastor Todd says an important part of recovery for any addict is to remove from your life everything that triggers it. If it's alcohol, get rid of all of it in your house. If it's a struggle for self-image, get rid of all your mirrors. If it's Internet pornography, break the computer. It's an extreme approach, but when your life is on the line, extremes are all you have.

So when Sarah confronted me that night, I grabbed a hammer, pulled the scales out of the closet, and hit them as I hard I could. I beat them until they were nothing but plastic pieces scattered across the yard. Seeing it that way, the scale didn't seem so powerful.

The constant fear of not knowing my weight didn't feel as heavy as I thought it would. I thought I would be consumed with it, kept up at night going crazy without knowledge of the number. Surprisingly, I found myself relieved. I see now it was all part of the devil's deception. He wants us to think the weight of life without our vices will be heavy when in fact, it's just the opposite. The weight of life lived in sin is heavier than any other.

It was the devil's deception that made me a slave to the number, but it was God's grace that started to set me free. I prayed, and I prayed hard. There were a lot of questions and even more tears. I begged God for His comfort every time I felt anxious about the scale. I pleaded for His strength to help me stay the course.

It's funny how debilitating the fear of the unknown can be. I was so afraid that not having the scale would make me crazy, but once I got rid of it, I saw that it was the scale that was making me crazy. I realized that my identity was not in a number on the scale; my identity was found in Christ and His approval of me. That's the truth addiction tries to take away from us. It takes away our identity. It makes us question who we really are. It makes us believe that we need it to survive. Ask any family member or friend of an addict about what it was like to see their loved one at the height of their addiction, and they'll all probably tell you some version of the same thing: that wasn't the person I knew. That's because addiction changes us.

Addiction isn't beat in one day. It's not over with one decision, one prayer, or one attempt at making it right. It takes time. The fear of gaining weight was still there. The pull of the scale still haunted me. The count of calories still sat in my mind. But this time, I was fighting back.

Without the scale I had to rely more on how I felt physically to gauge my health. Did I have enough energy to get through the day? Was I eating enough to fuel my body? It was hard to do, but I was trying to regain my life.

Of course there was still the question of running. I had to reshape my entire view of the sport. I had to hold on to what I loved about running--the joy, the freedom, the challenge--and let go of all the things I'd let it become--a punishment, an obligation, a means to an end.

I wanted to be able to run they way I used to before the disease but in order to get better I had to stop. I had to take a break. I had to focus on my health and then maybe running would happen again someday.

I wanted to be free.

Mile

24

Recovery

By 2014, I was on the road to recovery--the long, slow, difficult road to recovery. It had been about 6 months since I had been at my worst. I didn't know what recovery would look like, but it was initially defined as gaining weight. As I gained weight I began the process of finding myself again. I was allowing myself to eat, to put on weight slowly. Though it was hard to do, I was doing it. I did remember some of the advice given to me in my initial counseling sessions. My counselor told me to think about food like medicine. If I wanted to get better, I had to take my medicine.

Besides, if I wanted to live and possibly run again, I knew I had to eat. I hadn't run consistently for about four months at that point. I had hit rock bottom from a physical standpoint and knew that food was the starting point to getting my strength back. Slowly but surely I increased my calorie intake. And it was beginning to work. I felt better, my energy was up, and it seemed like I may actually be able to enjoy my life again.

That's not to say that my road wasn't full of setbacks. I was struggling against an array of mental setbacks every single day. I started running again once the weather warmed, and with that, I started making horrible eating choices again. I was basing them solely on calorie count, still calculating calories in and calories out. Something that became routine was a seven mile run in the morning and made sure to get in at least ten miles total before the day ended. My body didn't respond to running like it used to. My legs hurt, and I was much weaker. I was frustrated at this reality because I thought I would bounce back and adjust to running faster than this. Another toll of the disease on my life and how your body is affected by how it's fueled. If you don't put the proper nutrients into your body it will not function as best it can.

As I ran, my appetite increased. I started eating more, and as a result, started gaining weight. With every pound, Eddie was still there. He was still trying to hold me prisoner in my own mind. I was still binge eating, feeling guilty, and fighting the impulse to run away the guilt. I struggled back and forth with guilt and disappointment. I didn't want to overeat. I didn't want to be consumed with guilt and anxiety. The difference now was that at least I was fighting back. I was far from where I needed to be, but I was still trying.

Soon my brother signed up for a local half marathon, and I decided to go alongside him as a starting point to making running healthy again. Training and running with my brother felt like a safe way to start. I had no clue if I would be able to even finish it. My muscle mass, my strength, my stamina--they were all long gone. But I knew I wanted to try.

Part of trying meant eating. I had to eat to train. And I had to train if I wanted to run.

The morning of the race I woke up feeling like it was old times again. I got up early and had a big breakfast. As I ate, I noticed that I didn't feel the guilt and anxiety that had come with all of my breakfasts over the past year. With the race before me, I really was able to look at the food I ate that morning as fuel. That was one step closer to my end goal--to look at food as fuel all the time. I wasn't there yet, but this was a small win. Small wins are needed on the path to healing. You have to take the small wins like mile markers in a marathon; you aren't finished yet but don't quit. Keep going on the road to big wins.

On the way to the race that morning my brother asked me about my condition. I shared with him the details of my struggle, how I was still struggling but trying to get better. And I told him that this race felt like a step in the right direction.

I was nervous as we arrived, but as we walked to the start I was overcome with that race day euphoria all over again. I couldn't stop smiling. Something about being there just felt right.

I took my place in the back of the pack. There was no shame in that for me this day; I knew my goal was not to win, but to finish. That was victory enough for me. Each step I ran would be a step away from that person I had become. I didn't want to be consumed with calories. I didn't want to be a person that barely weighed enough to live. I wanted to be the Jesse who God created me to be.

As the race began, I was overcome with one thought: this is what I'm supposed to do. Everything felt right (except for that fall I took in the first mile over a road reflector. That felt wrong).

I started to play back the scenes of my life over the last eight months. The road to this point was painful, nasty, and tough. It was messy in every way. And even if the rest of this run were just as messy as the first mile, I would keep going. It was my road to recovery.

As my brother and I approached the third mile, my body was screaming for relief. My legs were really feeling it, and I realized just how tough finishing this thing was actually going to be. By mile five my brother and I were looking at each other like we were crazy. Whose idea was it to run this thing again?

By the time we got into mile six, I was in a steady stage of reflection. I was remembering how things used to be, what life looked like before this addiction. And I started to pray. I asked for God's forgiveness for everything I had done to my body. I apologized for losing sight of the way He created me in His image and for His purpose. I asked for help to continue to climb out of the pit of the devil's deception.

And before I knew it, we had hit mile nine. I might actually finish this thing! I called Sarah (who was hoping to meet me at the finish line) to give her our estimated time of arrival at the end. My brother was hoping to finish in 2:10, and I was trying my hardest to get there with him.

As we approached the finish line, the clock read 2:09. My brother broke off in a sprint to finish, leaving me in his dust! He had earned his time to celebrate at the finish line. And so had I.

As I crossed that finish line, I was overcome with gratitude. I was so thankful for the opportunity to run again, but even more grateful that I actually enjoyed it. Our family met us in excitement to celebrate the accomplishment.

For a moment, all felt right in the world.

Until someone suggested going out to eat in celebration.

Remember how I told you I was on the road to recovery? The messy, ugly, painful road? This is just one example of how ugly that road really is.

Eating still caused anxiety for me. I knew that wasn't going to just go away overnight. It would be a constant battle.

Even though I had just completed a run full of freedom and healing, I was still fighting against the lies in my mind.

Don't eat. Don't put those calories back. You'll only gain weight.

Sarah suggested I pick a place to eat. It shouldn't have been so hard. I was hungry and wanted to eat. Yet trying to pick a place that I actually thought would be good proved difficult. My anxiety over food combined with my weak and tired post-race state was the perfect storm for disaster.

I fought with Sarah there in the parking lot. It may be one of the only times we've actually yelled at one another. To this day, it remains one of the worst arguments we've ever had. I was angry at everything, frustrated with every word and suggestion from her. I've always wanted to treat Sarah the way she deserves to be treated. I want her to feel protected, loved, and provided for no matter what. But that day, I was failing miserably at all of those things, and all because of the mental battle I was waging in my mind over food.

Eventually I walked away from the conversation and headed to a local gas station. I sat down with a cup of coffee and collected my thoughts. I was embarrassed at my behavior. I was frustrated with myself for not being able to get myself together. I didn't want to be such a jerk, but I knew why I had been.

Addiction. Disease.

They were fighting hard for my mind in that moment, and I was letting them win.

Eventually I walked back to the car and apologized. I was wrong and embarrassed. As I look back now on events like these I'm reminded how strong of a woman I married. Sarah was then and still is committed to our vows, even during times when it would have been easier to walk away from them.

Recovery takes patience from family and friends. That's probably why my counselors suggested in-patient treatment to spare loved ones from the ugliness of the process. I wish I could tell you that days like this were few and far between, but that's just not the case. The devil and his deception didn't want to let go of me easily. Anxiety and anger were there waiting to creep back in every time my weight changed. They were there when I felt out of control about what to eat. They were there when I felt the urge to binge or run based on guilt.
It was a battle, and I was fighting it every minute of every day.

2014 was full of ups and downs, but it ultimately led me down the path to slowly getting better. I ran a full marathon in September of 2014, and remember calling my pastor Todd afterwards to celebrate.

"Hey man, I feel like I've got this disease whipped," I told him confidently. "I'm better now."

His response caught me off guard.

"Wait two years before you tell that to anyone," he simply said.

What did that mean? Why two years? It sounded extreme at the time, but looking back, I now know exactly what he meant. I was nowhere near where I needed to be. I was still fighting. One race meant winning a battle, but I was far from winning a war.

And so I pressed on.

Mile

25

Taking a toll

Anorexia certainly took a toll on my body. As I started to run again, I noticed my body didn't seem to feel or work the same way. I was extremely lethargic, mostly because of the food choices I was making. Looking back, I didn't need to be running. I viewed it as a sign of being one step closer to recovery--to the life I lived before disease. I wanted to be strong, energetic, and active. It was an internal struggle for me. I don't have much patience, and I wanted my old life back quickly. Full recovery takes a lot of time, and in order to keep going, I had to remind myself that just as my current condition didn't develop overnight, neither would my recovery.

So while I wanted to run as I used to all the time, my body was telling me to slow down and give it time. I would get blood work done every few months, and each time the results noted I was anemic. My vitamin levels were always low as well. I couldn't understand that I wasn't eating the right kinds of food to aid my body in recovering physically. This is why professional help is so very important. I

150

couldn't do it on my own because I didn't know how to feed my body correctly. I learned to rely on the expertise and advice from medical professionals who only wanted the best for me.

The end of 2014 and the beginning of 2015 were full of distractions, distractions in a helpful way. I started to use other things to take my mind off food. I put myself in environments where I felt comfortable and safe in order to divert my mind from obsessing over food choices. And believe it or not, it started to work. My energy level increased and so did my ability to focus on things other than food.

By August of 2015 I began to research and attend counseling sessions again. I began to listen to medical professionals on what to do. I constantly had to remind Eddie that was I was doing was helping my body by eating. I also constantly reminded myself that I needed to listen to the people in my life who were trying to help me. Even when I didn't want to, I needed to say, "Okay." That was a big part of the healing process for me. Total surrender. I had to develop the discipline of eating what was in front of me, hungry or not. I had to say okay to the food choices given to me. If my counselor suggested not to run for a few weeks, I had to say okay. It was one word, but a big act of full surrender on my part.

But it was the birth of my third child that really got my attention. Grady was born in October 2015. Everything went as planned and he was brought into the world early in the morning. However, while the nurses were cleaning him up, they kept cheering him on and telling him to breathe. I didn't understand what was happening, as I hadn't heard this with the birth of my first two children. Eventually we were informed that Grady needed to be placed on oxygen and kept in the nursery. They let us take one last look and then rushed him to the nursery.

Over the course of the day, things worsened quickly. He was transported to a nearby children's hospital and placed in a room to be monitored. At only one day old, he was being monitored by nine machines, all-working to help him breathe. It was such a blur. Sarah was still at the other hospital eagerly waiting to be discharged and so I split my time between her and our son.

One specific conversation I had with a nurse truly changed my life. Grady was breathing about 160 reps a minute, with his heart beating nearly just as fast.

"How long can he keep breathing that fast?" I asked the nurse.

She responded honestly. "I'm not sure. Our bodies can only take so much before they just give out."

I was startled at her honesty at first, but as I thought about her words over the next few hours, it was as if God was speaking to me through her. I was destroying my body, and her words rang loud and clear. *Our bodies can only take so much before they just give out.* Grady hadn't done anything to his body, and yet he was suffering. Yet I was sitting there praying for his healing while destroying my own body with my choices.

That night was a turning point. I wanted to be healthy. I wanted to be there for Grady--for all my kids. I wanted to do all I could to spearhead my recovery to lead a long and healthy life for my children. I've never audibly heard the voice of God but in that hospital room I heard the message loud and clear. I had to get better. What seemed so important for so long, the necessity to be skinny, couldn't matter any less.

I was ready to work.

Thankfully, Grady recovered, and now, I wanted to as well. I wanted to get better, and food was the medicine to help me. I had to make sure I ate what I needed to be healthy. That's when I began the refeeding process. I would continue to slowly increase my calories and the types of food that I ate over an extended period of time. It was a slow start to gaining weight and making healthy choices.

Surprisingly, the refeeding process made my central nervous system go haywire! I started having constant muscle twitches all over my body, but especially in my legs. I experienced extreme cramps overnight, telling Sarah that I'd wake up feeling as though I'd run ten miles during the night. Over the course of the next six months, I saw doctors almost on a weekly basis to figure out what damage had been done to my body. I went through a battery of testing--blood work, MRI's, CT scans, the works! Each one brought with it an extreme amount of guilt. Had I not made terrible choices, my body wouldn't be suffering the way it was now. Counseling helped me navigate those feelings of guilt, recognizing them as the influence of Eddie in my mind.

It was the combination of those doctors, my counselor, and a professional nutritionist that helped me understand that my body was suffering because I wasn't feeding it what it needed. I remember being shocked when a nutritionist told me that my brain needed 60 grams of fat each day to function properly. I was shocked. How does someone eat 60 grams of fat a day?! I mean, I KNOW how but to actually eat that much was going to be tough. But I knew she was right and I had to listen. Consulting with professionals like her helped me understand what I needed to put in my body and mind to be healthy. I can't stress enough how helpful my counselors, and doctors were. I would plead with anyone struggling with an eating disorder or addiction to seek the help of a professional. Don't try to do it on your own.

It was January of 2016 when I went to the doctor and saw the scale read 165. I had gained 30 pounds since Grady's birth. I laughed as the nurse looked at the scale as though it was broken. I knew it was right, and for the first time in a long time, I was glad it was right. A higher number meant a healthier Jesse. And because I was feeding my body the right way, I knew a bigger number was a good sign.

My counselor was right. I had to get back to a certain weight in order for my mind to start working again. It's a different number for everyone, but for me, it was about 155 pounds. Once I hit that mark, I started to view food in a healthier way. The desire to binge wasn't there. The urge to restrict wasn't there either. For the first time in years, I felt normal. And that felt great.

There's nothing easy about overcoming a disease like anorexia. It's certainly not quick, and life after rarely goes back to the way it was. Instead, you learn to embrace a new normal.

My new normal included a lot of different things to help me sustain my recovery. For starters, it took accountability. I had to surround myself with people who would ask me tough questions and demand honest answers. They never hesitated to ask about running, how much and how often I was doing it. They asked me about eating and weighing. They knew all of my triggers and boldly asked about each one of them to help me avoid a downward spiral. Their accountability helped give my recovery sustainability.

Another part of my recovery was seeking professional help. As hard as it might have been to admit, I knew I needed an expert's guidance to stay on the right path. My counselor understood my condition inside and out and was able to provide me with the tools I needed to recover. She was a safe place to vent, someone who would listen without bias and give me the advice I needed to stay on track. With her help I was able to identify my fears and learn how long Eddie had truly been impacting my life. Counseling was then and still is crucial to the success of my recovery.

My family was an incredible part of my recovery. I can't say enough about all my wife did for me throughout this struggle. She started fighting for my recovery before I even knew I needed it. She encouraged and supported me-- even when I failed her. She deserved none of what the disease caused our family, but she never walked away. The same can be said for the rest of my family. My children, my parents, my brother--none of them deserved the way I treated them or the consequences of the disease in their lives. Yet they never let that get in the way of supporting me.

My relationship with God and all it included--prayer, church, spending time with Him--were precious to me during and after my recovery. Church allowed me to engage with other families in safe, uplifting environment. Very few knew the details of my condition, making it a place where I could feel free from the weight of addiction. It brought me so much comfort just to be in the company of other believers.

Surrender. This was the key for me. It had to happen daily and still does. I had to surrender when I was 112 pounds, and I still do at 160 pounds. I have to lay down control. When a counselor, medical professional, or accountability partner would tell me not to run or suggest a meal option, I had to surrender to their advice and know it was what was best. Though at times I felt like a puppet on a string, it was necessary to give up my control in order to get it back in a healthy, balanced way. I had to put my life in someone else's hands until I could manage it without destruction.

Often, addicts and those struggling with disease believe the lie that we are alone. Addiction separates us from everyone else, and at times, we even prefer it that way. But in recovery, you have to break free of that lie in order to fight. You can't fight alone. In the times I felt most alone, I would pray. Sometimes I didn't even know what to pray. In those moments, I would just utter one question to God: how? How was I going to survive this? How was I going to get my life back? How would I be able to keep up recovery? And even though God didn't give me all the answers I wanted, I knew He was there.

As for that question of how, I can answer that myself now. I answer it by not running. I answer it by turning to God. I answer it by eating balanced and avoiding a binge. If I feel an impulse to not eat, I combat it with healthy things like prayer and counseling rather than giving in or running. They help me keep my eyes on the road to recovery and silence the voice of Eddie.

What I learned in the fight for my life is that the devil's deception is only powerful until you listen to God. His voice is louder, stronger, and much more powerful than any lie the devil has to tell. And with God, I have the ultimate tools I need to win the fight. I just have to use them.

I often feel like Peter, being asked to step out of the boat in the middle of a storm. Jesus was standing ahead of him on the rough waters, beckoning Peter towards him. Yet the idea of getting out the boat was almost paralyzing to Peter. It took courage and faith to take just that first step. But he took it. And guess what? He didn't drown. Why? Because he put his complete faith and surrender in Jesus to keep him alive.

I'm trying to do the same, one step at a time.

Mile

26

I actually can finish!

Looking back, I now know what the problem really was. I found my confidence and security in the numbers, opinions, and others. I believed they were the most accurate evaluation of my condition and the person I was. I looked to them for validation when I should have been looking to the God who created me and gave me life.

I put my identity in what I could do instead of the person I was. It's an unhealthy way to live. God created each of us uniquely, and in order to keep going, we have to be confident in the way He created us. We can't worry about other people's perceptions. When we chase someone else's idea of perfection, we'll surely be miserable. But when we look to God, we find rest.

I now define recovery as finding something that was lost. I lost my identity in anorexia. I lost my identity in the numbers. And in order to recover, I had to find who I really was--the person God created me to be. When I did that, working on the rest didn't seem so overwhelming.

Looking back, I see how early the seeds of lies were planted in my mind. Overweight as a child and struggling to fit in taught me to look for my confidence in anything other than myself. Initially I found it in running. It allowed me to prove myself, working hard to see the results I wanted. When the numbers on the clock or the number on the scale were lower, I felt confident. I felt accomplished.

And, on its own, that doesn't have to be a bad thing! Setting and accomplishing goals is a great habit, but the fault comes in believing those accomplishments bring worth. My fault came when I allowed myself to believe that everything in my life hinged on the numbers.

My confidence should have come from God. I'd heard it time and again from the Bible. *We are fearfully and wonderfully made.* Now, I really understand it. My worth and wonder is in being God's creation. He created me with a unique and specific purpose, and He wants to use me exactly as I am. I'm not the same as everyone else, but that's a strength, not a hindrance.

Today, I can tell you that my confidence lies in who I am in Christ, how much He loves and cares for me just the way I am, and how I'm using who I am to make an impact on the world for His glory.

And more than anything, I want you to see yourself the same way. You are created by God. You are special. You are unique. And you have an incredible potential just exactly as you are right now. Leverage your uniqueness to make an impact on the lives of those around you. Be confident in who you are in Christ and follow Him down the road to your best life.

That's a race worth running.

.2

The last .2 of the race is up to you. You have to decide what you really want and pursue the help you need to get there. Recovery is possible but it requires more than just willpower. Don't allow the lies of the devil to tell you anything different. Don't follow him down a road that will stop you from being the person God made you to be. I speak from experience when I tell you that the only thing you'll find at the end of that road is disappointment, darkness, and maybe even death.

When you follow the road God has laid out before you, there's so much more ahead than you can even imagine. Trust me, I would know!

So make the last .2 count. Step out of the boat and start running towards the life God has for you. The last .2 takes trust. I had to trust those put in place for my recovery. I had to trust they knew what they were doing and wanted the best for me. Recovery is great and attainable but it is a long road with many small steps. A marathon is 26.2 different miles that require different amounts of effort that make up one long race. There are many small steps in getting to the finish line. All of them have been full of emotion and dedicated work. Keep moving forward.

Recovery is tough, but it's worth it.